Exploring Galena and Dubuque on Foot

David Ryan

Exploring Galena and Dubuque on Foot

By Sidewalk, Stairway, and Path

By David Ryan

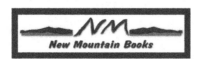

New Mountain Books
Albuquerque, New Mexico

....

Dedication

This book is dedicated to my
Galena ancestors and their descendants.

....

First Edition 2020
10 9 8 7 6 5 4 3 2 1
Library of Congress Control Number: 2020932932
ISBN: 978-0-9776968-5-7
Disclaimer – New Mountain Books and the author assume no liability for
accidents happening to, or injuries sustained by, readers who engage in activities
described in this book.

Photographs: All photographs by David Ryan except where noted.
Cover and book design by Mark Sullivan
Typefaces: Adobe Caslon Pro and Barlow

Published By:
New Mountain Books
Albuquerque, New Mexico
www.newmountainbooks.com

Table of Contents

Preface

This book, *Exploring Galena and Dubuque on Foot*, is a series of walking tours through two of the most scenic communities in the entire country! Very few people outside of the Midwest are aware of the area's natural beauty or of its cultural and historical significance. On top of that Galena and Dubuque are two amazing communities to explore. Especially on foot!

The tours in this book are designed to get you out of the car and to go at a pace that allows you to observe. When you begin to observe, you'll be amazed at all of the little details that pop out and grab your attention. They in turn will take you in directions that you never imagined. And while walking, you'll also have the opportunity to find quietude. Rather than overwhelming noise and stimulation, you'll have the chance to hear sounds. Sounds of church bells, birds, footsteps, or just quiet.

The title of this book could have easily been reversed to *Exploring Dubuque and Galena on Foot*. I chose the sequence of Galena first for two reasons. One is that Galena was settled first. And the other is that I personally have roots in Galena. All of my Irish ancestors (and my last name) came from Galena. I even have two grandparents, an aunt, and many of their predecessors buried in Galena.

As for the walks, our first one explores the places that were turning points in the life of Ulysses S. Grant. Although Grant only lived full-time in Galena for the year just before the Civil War, he would not have had the opportunity to become the general who won the Civil

War and then went on to become president if he had not lived in Galena for that one year!

Our second walk in Galena explores the town's historic core that includes the finest collection of buildings from the 1840s and 1850s in the country. The walk takes advantage of Galena's many stairways that connect the center of town to the homes high above on the bluffs. Our third walk is west of Galena in East Dubuque, Illinois. There we'll explore the best preserved Native-American burial mounds in the area.

In Dubuque we have four walks exploring the neighborhoods above and below the bluffs west and northwest of downtown Dubuque. Along the way we'll ride a funicular (incline railway), climb several stairways, walk through what is perhaps the highest concentration of late Victorian homes in the country, and discover many other surprises!

Our fifth and final walk in Dubuque checks out several Native-American burial mounds on a wooded bluff north of town, an amazing view of the Mississippi River from Eagle Point Park, and a hike up to the Julien Dubuque monument south of town.

With that, I'm sure that you'll agree that Galena and Dubuque are very special communities and wonderful places to explore on foot.

Chapter One

Galena and Dubuque

Galena, Illinois and Dubuque, Iowa are only sixteen miles apart on U.S. Highway 20 and located where the states of Iowa, Wisconsin, and Illinois come together in the Upper Mississippi River Valley. With the broad river, lush valleys, tall hills, and rugged rock-faced bluffs, it is one of the prettiest places in the country! If your only impression of the Midwest has been a drive on Interstate 80 or a visit to Chicago, you will be shocked by the natural beauty of the Upper Mississippi River Valley. In addition to a wonderful natural setting there is an abundance of history and, perhaps, the greatest concentration of 19th-century buildings in the country.

Along with their scenic settings, both communities are great places to be. Dubuque has been designated an "All American City" multiple times and was most recently designated in 2019. The Galena area is a popular visitor destination and second home location, and many publications have named Galena the best this, or the prettiest that, or the nicest small town in America.

With their core areas developed in the 19th century when people got around by public transportation or on foot, Galena and Dubuque were meant to be walked. With historic buildings and scenic views almost everywhere, there are plenty of nooks and crannies to check out and explore. And with stairways to navigate the hills and relatively short blocks providing plenty of places to make turns, it is easy to get around on foot.

The Driftless

The natural beauty of Galena and Dubuque comes from being at the southern tip of "the Driftless." The Driftless is land that was missed by the glaciers of the most recent Ice Ages and encompasses the southeast corner of Minnesota, southwestern Wisconsin, the northeastern edge of Iowa, and the far northwest corner of Illinois. The name Driftless comes from the absence of glacial drift (or deposits). There is some evidence that earlier Ice Age flows did leave glacial drift in the Iowa portion of the Driftless. As a point of reference, the most recent ice flows left Illinois around 16,000 years ago.

The varied topography of the Driftless comes from the land not being bulldozed flat by Ice Age glaciers. So whatever preconceived impression you may have of Midwestern topography, it does not apply to the Driftless. Rather than the flat or gently rolling countryside normally associated with much of the Midwest, the Driftless has readily identifiable topography of tall hills (oftentimes called mounds), deep valleys, and rock-faced bluffs. Charles Mound at 1,235 feet of elevation is Illinois' highest point and is only 15 miles or so from Galena.[1]

In an earlier geologic time (more than 300 million years ago) the interior of the country was a shallow sea. As a result most of the rock in the Driftless is a form of sedimentary limestone, sandstone, or shale. The predominant bedrock in the Galena and Dubuque area is limestone and dolomite. Dolomite is very similar to limestone. The bedrock is also very close to the surface.

Also in an earlier geologic time (250 million years ago or so), the sedimentary rock was uplifted to form a plateau. There is some belief

---

1. If you are a state highpointer and want to walk to Illinois' highpoint, Charles Mound is privately owned and only open on the first full weekends of June, July, August, and September. Dogs are not allowed. Please inquire first to check on any changes.

that the higher elevations of the plateau caused the Ice Age glaciers to go around the area rather than over it. Over time, the normal course of erosion carved deep valleys and hills. The prominent peaks (or mounds) are located where the rock was the hardest.

At some point during this time an igneous (volcanic) event, probably in the form of a superheated mineral-rich brine, bought up mineral matter (primarily lead) from the interior of the earth. The brine penetrated the creases and crevices of the sedimentary rock and left rich veins of mineral ore. And since the Ice Age glaciers did not plow through the Driftless, the ore was left in place and not carried away. And it was this presence of lead that brought the first European-American settlers to the area.

Lead Mining

With an abundance of lead outcrops, Native Americans were the first to dig lead out of the ground to make paint and to use as a trade good. Early French explorers and voyageurs traded with local tribes for lead. One French Canadian from Quebec, Julien Dubuque, obtained permission in 1788 from local tribes to mine lead just south of today's Dubuque. The City of Dubuque is, of course, named after him. At that time, the land west of the Mississippi River was nominally a Spanish possession and Dubuque named his enterprise "Mines of Spain."

European-American settlement and mining did not arrive in the Galena area until the 1820s. Even though a specific location may have been in a territory or a state of the United States, a location was not open to European-American settlement or commercial development until the United States government negotiated treaties with the local Native-American tribes. Dubuque which is Iowa's oldest city, on the other side of the Mississippi River, was not open to settlers until the 1830s. The entire three state region of Galena, Dubuque, and southwestern Wisconsin experienced a huge lead mining boom in the 1830s and 1840s. The City of Galena was named after the lead mineral of galena.

Galena Becomes the Commercial Center of the Mining District

Before railroads and paved highways, rivers were the preferred method of travel. With Galena's location on the Fever River (later renamed the Galena River) three and a half miles upriver from the Mississippi River, Galena became the largest river port between St. Louis and St. Paul. This made Galena the commercial hub for a region that extended into Iowa, Minnesota, and Wisconsin. The combination of mining, riverboats, and regional commerce produced substantial wealth for Galena. As a result many fine homes and commercial establishments were built in Galena during the 1840s and 1850s.

When the Illinois Central Railroad reached Galena in 1854, Galena was intended to be the western terminus of the railroad. But because the City of Galena and the railroad could not agree upon where to build the railroad terminal in Galena, the Illinois Central obtained permission to continue the line west beyond Galena to Dunleith (today's East Dubuque) on the Mississippi River. The railroad reached Dunleith in 1855 and finally crossed the Mississippi River into Dubuque when the railroad bridge was opened in 1869.

By the time the railroad reached Galena, lead mining was already beginning to be played out and the Galena River was starting to silt up. With mines digging into the earth, plows turning over the land for farms, and trees being cut to provide fuel for lead smelting, there wasn't enough of the original prairie vegetation to keep the soil from running off and silting up the Galena River. With riverboating and mining in decline, Galena's population peaked in 1858 at 14,000 and then began a steady drop. Galena's role as a regional center was further reduced when the Civil War disrupted river travel and made railroads the dominant means to move people and freight.

Galena's New Reality

Galena did not disappear, but it no longer dominated regional commerce. It transitioned to a local agricultural hub with some locally based industries. But with all the farm land claimed and increasing mechanization reducing the need for agricultural labor, Galena did not have enough economic activity to support its earlier population levels. By 1900 Galena's population was down to 5,000. Today's (2020) population is now around 3,200.

With fewer people and no prospects for growth there wasn't any pressure on Galena to bulldoze its commercial center to make room for new construction. Nor did it need to make way for shopping malls, office towers, or parking decks. Galena did not have to clear out neighborhoods to make room for new housing. Instead Galena took a break and left everything as it was.

And it's a good thing. Over time, people woke up to the fact that tucked into an extraordinarily scenic valley in the far northwest corner of Illinois was the finest collection of 1840s and 1850s buildings in the country. And even better, there were plenty of Galena residents who also recognized the value of what they had and did their part to protect it. Today over 85% of the community is listed in the National Register of Historic Places.

And if Galena's most famous resident, Ulysses S. Grant, were to come back today for a visit he would still recognize where he was. And what's even better is that Galena is the real deal. It is not a reconstructed Williamsburg nor a Disney-like theme park; it is a real living community that is a great place to reside or to visit for a nice getaway. And even better, it's a fantastic place to explore on foot!

Dubuque

As Iowa's oldest city, Dubuque, too, has much to offer. Not only as a place to live but also as a place to visit. And like Galena, Dubuque is a fantastic place to explore on foot.

In 1850, Galena was quite a bit bigger than Dubuque, but by 1860, Dubuque was starting to pull ahead. Whereas Galena took a break, Dubuque continued to grow and to participate in the national economy. With a population today (2020) of around 58,000, Dubuque is not a big city but it is a diverse and complete city with a mixed economy, colleges, museums, and plenty of activities. With it right on the Mississippi River and surrounded by bluffs Dubuque is in an extremely attractive setting. Whereas Galena has an abundance of buildings from the 1840s and 1850s, Dubuque has an extraordinarily large concentration of late Victorian homes and buildings.

Dubuque, like Galena, got its start with lead mining. And like Galena, lead mining eventually ran its course in Dubuque. But unlike Galena, other industries came to take its place. In the second half of the 19th century and in the first part of the 20th century, Dubuque's location on the Mississippi River combined with its multiple rail connections made it an important lumber and wood products center.

During the second half of the 19th century, the Upper Midwest was the center of the logging industry. Logs were cut in northeastern Minnesota and northwestern Wisconsin during the winter and dragged down to major tributaries of the Mississippi. In the spring when the rivers thawed, the logs were assembled into huge log rafts and floated down the Mississippi River to downstream sawmills. Several towns along the Mississippi, including Dubuque, had large mills to process the logs into lumber and into finished wood products. With railroads going in every direction from Dubuque, the finished wood products were easily distributed to the end user. When the forests of the Upper Midwest ran out of timber, large scale logging moved to other parts of the country and the age of the large sawmills along the Mississippi came to an end.

As industries have come and gone, Dubuque has continued to thrive. The legacy of the fortunes made in the 19th century can be still be found in the form of magnificent houses in the bluffs and on the streets of Dubuque. We'll be passing many of them as we explore Dubuque on foot!

Exploring Galena and Dubuque on Foot

This book is first and foremost about walking and exploring. It is organized around several different walks in Galena, East Dubuque, and Dubuque. The walks within Galena and Dubuque proper are in areas that were developed at a time when people traveled around on foot or relied upon public transportation. The walks are in walkable neighborhoods.

Walkable communities have houses built close to each other to make it easier to reach a neighbor on foot. When houses are closer to each other there is a sense of mass and an abundance of details that make the neighborhood more interesting, especially to those on foot. Walkable communities have a grid pattern of streets or a sufficient number of cross streets to make it easier to reach a neighbor living on a nearby street. Walkable communities located in hilly areas often-times have public stairways to provide a direct route to streets at a higher or lower elevation. And the ultimate walkable community has stores, schools, and services within reasonable walking distance.

The walks in this book take advantage of public stairways, side-walks, and paths wherever possible to explore hidden corners and to seek out items of interest and other surprises along the way.

History does play a role in some of the walks, but this book is not a comprehensive regional history. This book is about what you can find and experience today. This book does point out many interesting buildings along the way, but again this is not a comprehensive historical architectural guide to the region. The narrative does not get bogged down with information on who the architect was or who built the house. The book sometimes does mention who lived in a particular house when relevant.

This book is not a walking tour of downtown Dubuque or a guide to every Dubuque neighborhood. This book focuses on neighborhoods with bluffs, stairways, and walkable streets.

The main purpose of the book is to get you out and to start exploring. The walks described in the book are meant to give you an idea of what's available. You are welcome to modify a walk in any way you see fit, and once you start exploring, you'll be amazed at all that you'll notice and discover.

Architectural Style References

Although this is not a comprehensive architectural guide, the book oftentimes notes the architectural style of a building. The styles mentioned in this book include:

Federal Style – On the East Coast, Federal-style buildings are from 1780 to 1830. In Galena, they are from the 1840s and 1850s. A Federal-style building is typically a two room deep brick building with a symmetrical arrangement of windows that oftentimes have shutters and small panes of glass. Depending upon the size of the house, the front door will be in the center or located where one of the symmetrical windows should be. Ulysses S. Grant's pre-Civil War Galena home is a good example of a Federal-style building.

Italianate Style – An Italianate-style building generally, but not always, has a low-pitched roof with eaves supported by intricate corbels. Windows can have majestic looking treatments called pediments. Some Italianate-style buildings will have cupolas on the roof. Ulysses S. Grant's post-Civil War Galena house is an example of an Italianate-style house.

Greek Revival Style – A Greek Revival building has large columns and looks like a Greek temple from the front. The Elihu Washburne house in Galena is good example of a Greek Revival house.

Second Empire Style – Second Empire is named for Napoleon III of France (1850s-70s). Buildings typically feature mansard roofs, ornamentation, and oftentimes looks like something from the French Renaissance. An example of a Second Empire building is at 605 Bluff Street in Dubuque.

Queen Anne Style – Queen Anne-style houses in America were built from 1880 to 1910 and are what most of us think of as Victorian. They are usually asymmetrical, have over-hanging eaves with a dominant front-facing gable, towers, and porches. Dubuque has an abundance of Queen Anne-style houses.

Gothic Revival Style – A Gothic Revival building has a vertical emphasis with steep pitched roofs and pointed arches and windows. They are irregular in appearance and have plenty of decoration. A good example of a Gothic Revival house is at 1207 Grove Terrace in Dubuque.

Richardsonian Romanesque Style – Richardsonian Romanesque is named after the architect Henry Hobson Richardson. The style was popular from 1880 to 1900. The buildings are always made from heavy stone and have elaborate window and door treatments. A good example of a Richardsonian Romanesque home is at 1105 Locust Street in Dubuque.

Craftsman Style – Craftsman-style homes were very popular in the early 20th century. Because our walks tend to go through areas developed in the 19th century, we will not be passing many Craftsman homes. Craftsman homes are simple and are oftentimes called bungalows. They tend to emphasize the horizontal rather than the vertical and have low-pitched roofs with pronounced overhanging eaves and exposed beams. They can also have porches and artistic decorations. We will pass a Craftsman home at 1051 Walnut Street in Dubuque.

Art Deco / Art Moderne Style – Art Deco and Art Moderne styles apply more to commercial buildings than to residences. They are sleek buildings from the 1920s and 30s with distinctive designs. The Telegraph-Herald Building and the Historic Federal Building in Dubuque are examples of Art Deco / Art Moderne Style.

Public Stairways

In addition to being a book about exploring, this book is also a comprehensive guide to the public stairways of Galena and Dubuque. Since both communities have steep bluffs and hilly settings, public stairways were necessary to get from the top of the hill down to the bottom. Ulysses S. Grant took stairs to get from his pre-Civil War house in Galena at the top of the bluff down to his work, his church, and almost everywhere else he had to be in town.

With people now getting around by car, several of the public stairways in Galena and Dubuque have been removed. Fortunately for us, the stairways that do remain today play a critical role in their respective town's transportation infrastructure and are likely to remain.

Since stairways are such an amazing way to explore a neighborhood, the walks in this book have incorporated the following stairways:

Galena Stairways

Name of Stairway	Number of Steps*	Chapter(s)	Comment
Veterans Memorial Park Steps	85	3	Very Nice / Special
Magazine Street Steps	78	3	A Very Special Portal to a Great Walk
Winery Parking Lot Steps	54	3	Convenient
Warren Street Steps	46	3	Convenient
Green Street - High School Steps	149	3	Spectacular / Must Do!
Washington Street Steps	252	2, 3	Spectacular / Must Do!
Hill Street Steps	92	3	A Very Special Portal to a Great Walk
Perry Street	18 / 19	3	Has Other Values Besides the Steps
Old Jail Steps	88	3	A Great Place to Explore
Van Buren Street Steps	105	2	A Great Way to Reach the Grant House
Third Street Steps	30	2	Convenient
Einsweiler Bridge Steps	36	2, 3	Convenient
Levee Steps	24 / 32/ 31	2, 3	Convenient
Madison Street Steps	100+	3	Closed

East Dubuque Stairways

Name of Stairway	Number of Steps*	Chapter(s)	Comment
Jordan Avenue to Gramercy Park	125	4	A Very Special Portal to a Great Site
Gramercy Park	69	4	A Good Place to Explore

Dubuque Stairways

Name of Stairway	Number of Steps*	Chapter(s)	Comment
5th Street Steps	127	5	A Great Connection from Downtown
Hill Street to 7th Street Steps	60	5	Very Nice
8th Street Steps	35	5	Convenient with an Interesting Wall
11th Street Steps	173	6	These Stairs are Magical! / Must Do!
Loras to Montrose Terrace Steps	28	6	Convenient
Bluff to Montrose Terrace Steps	87	6	Very Nice and Very Pretty
Little Maquoketa River Mounds	120	9	A Special Portal to a Great Site
Mines of Spain	50	9	A Convenient Portal to a Great Site
West Locust to Catherine Steps	100+	6	Closed
West Locust to Hodgden Steps	100+	6	Closed

*All step counts are subject to being off a step or two due to miscounting.

A Note About Maps and Directions for Galena and Dubuque

The map of Galena on page 14 applies to both of the Galena chapters. Each Dubuque proper chapter has its own map.

For the purpose of directions, the streets of Galena tend to conform to the arc of the Galena River. This means that the actual direction of an east-west street or north-south street may be a little different than the direction given in the walk descriptions.

In Dubuque, many of the streets conform to the shape of a nearby bluff. Again this may result in an actual direction of a street being a little different than the direction given in the walk descriptions.

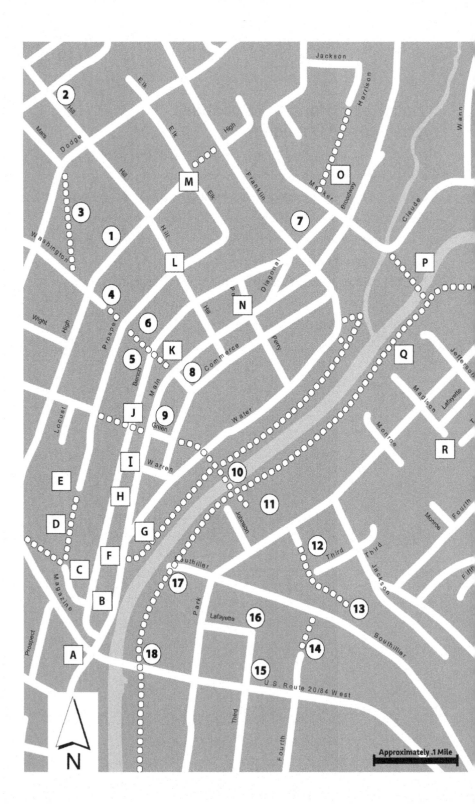

The Walking Tour of Ulysses S. Grant's Galena (Chapter 2) begins at his Pre-Civil War Home (Location 1). All location refences for the Grant tour are numbers in circles.

The Walking Tour through the Heart of Galena (Chapter 3) begins at the intersection of Spring and Main (Location A). All location references for the Heart of Galena tour are letters in squares.

Dotted Lines are pedestrian passages.

1. Ulysses S. Grant's Pre-Civil War Home (121 S. High Street)
2. John Rawlins and William Rowley Homes (517 and 515 Hill Street)
3. Old City Cemetery and Park
4. Top of the Washington Street Steps (Down)
5. 1851 Firehouse; the Galena and U.S. Grant Museum is just to the south (211 S. Bench)
6. Grant's Church and Pew; First United Methodist Church (125 S. Bench)
7. Jo Daviess County Courthouse
8. Grant Leather Store (122 S. Main in the Coatsworth Building)
9. DeSoto House Hotel (Northeast Corner of Main and Green Streets)
10. Pedestrian Bridge over the Galena River
11. Grant Park
12. Van Buren Street Steps (Up)
13. Ulysses S. Grant Post-Civil War Home
14. 4th Street Path
15. Elihu Washburne House
16. Steps Down to Playground Park
17. 1857 Galena Train Station
18. Steps Up to Frank Einsweiler Bridge and Pedestrian Walkway

A. Intersection of Spring (U.S. Highway 20) and Main Streets
B. Veterans Memorial Park Steps
C. Galena Public Library
D. Magazine Street Steps
E. Linmar Gardens
F. Galena Flood Gates
G. Levee Path
H. Winery Parking Lot Steps
I. Warren Street Steps
J. Green Street / High School Steps
K. Washington Street Steps
L. Hill Street Steps
M. Sidewalk Passage Between High and Franklin Streets
N. Perry Street
O. Old Jail Steps
P. Meeker Street Pedestrian Bridge
Q. Galena River Trail
R. Madison Street Steps

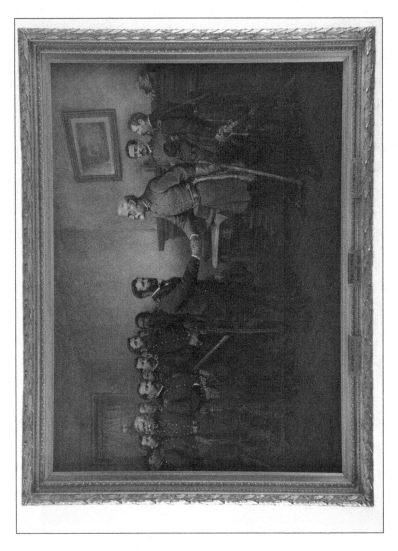

Peace in the Union by Thomas Nast- Courtesy of the Galena-Jo Daviess County Historical Society

Chapter Two

A Walking Tour of Ulysses S. Grant's Galena

Although Ulysses S. Grant did not move to Galena until one year before the Civil War, he would not have achieved the fame and success that we know him for had he not moved to Galena. This walk encompasses those places and events that made it possible for Ulysses S. Grant to win the Civil War and then go on to become President. The walk begins at his pre–Civil War home high above downtown Galena and visits all the sites that impacted his life while in Galena.

As one of the most prominent figures in U.S. history, Ulysses S. Grant is without a doubt Galena's most famous resident. Grant moved to Galena one year before the Civil War and was only an occasional and part-time resident after the war. But if he had not spent that year prior to the Civil War in Galena, it is highly unlikely that he would have become the Civil War general who won the war and then went on to become the 18th President of the United States!

After many years of unfavorable treatment by some historians, Grant's legacy is now looked upon more favorably.[1] After all it was his strategy and persistence that won the Civil War. And it was his presidency that made a serious effort to protect the rights of and to improve the lot of the former slaves. It wasn't until after World War II

---

1. *Grant* by Ron Chernow (published 2017) is an excellent biography of Grant.

during the Civil Rights era that other presidencies would even come close the Grant presidency in doing something about discrimination against and the second-class citizenship of the African-American community.

And it is for these reasons that it is worthwhile to walk around to see the places that affected Ulysses S. Grant's life during his time in Galena.

Ulysses S. Grant came to Galena because he was at the lowest point of his life, and as Robert Frost reminded us in his poem *Death of the Hired Man*:

> 'Home is the place where, when you have to go there,
> They have to take you in.'

At the beginning of 1860, West Point graduate, Mexican War veteran, and former U.S. Army captain, Ulysses S. Grant, was lost. He had been forced to leave the Army in the spring of 1854 because the separation from his family and the isolation of frontier Army posts drove him into a deep depression which led him to finding solace in a bottle.

After leaving the Army, Grant tried to make a go of it in the St. Louis area where his wife, Julia Dent Grant, was raised. Every enterprise from farming to business that he attempted failed. Those five years in Missouri were so painful for him that Grant devoted only three paragraphs to them in his *Personal Memoirs*.[2]

In debt and with nowhere else to turn, he turned to his father from whom he had been trying to get away ever since he left Ohio

---

2. Grant wrote his *Personal Memoirs* late in his life when he had been wiped out financially by a dishonest business associate and knew he was dying. With help from his friend Mark Twain, he wrote his memoirs to provide for his family financially after he died. Grant finished writing the memoirs just before he died. The book is exceptionally well written and was an instant success. It has never gone out of print.

for West Point in 1839. Grant's father, Jesse R. Grant, then lived in Covington, Kentucky (across the Ohio River from Cincinnati) and had a successful leather business with tanneries in Ohio and stores in Wisconsin, Iowa, and Galena, Illinois. A leather business in 1860 was not a leather shop selling purses and wallets as you might expect to find in a shopping mall of today. An 1860 leather business dealt in saddles, harnesses, leather for making boots and the like, and also would have dealt in hides to be tanned.

The store in Galena was run by Grant's two younger brothers (Simpson and Orvil) and served customers in Illinois, Iowa, Minnesota, and Wisconsin. Simpson, who had built the Galena business, was suffering from tuberculosis. As a result, Jesse offered Ulysses a job as a clerk in the Galena store paying $600 a year working for his two younger brothers.

With all other options exhausted, Captain Grant at the age of 38 accepted the position. He and his family boarded the steamboat *Itasca* in St. Louis for the four-day voyage to Galena in April 1860.

Ironically, thirteen months later, Henry David Thoreau (author of *Walden*) also boarded the *Itasca*. He was on a trip west to seek relief from tuberculosis. His travels took him by train to Dunleith (today's East Dubuque, Illinois) only a few miles from Galena on the Mississippi River. There he boarded the *Itasca* for the three-day voyage to St. Paul. After two months of travel, Thoreau, still suffering from tuberculosis, returned to Massachusetts where he died less than a year later in May 1862.

Although it has been 160 years since Captain Grant came to Galena, there is still a lot that he would recognize. To tour Grant's Galena we'll start our walk at his pre-Civil War home at 121 S. High Street. This is a good place to begin as street parking is very easy to find in this part of town.

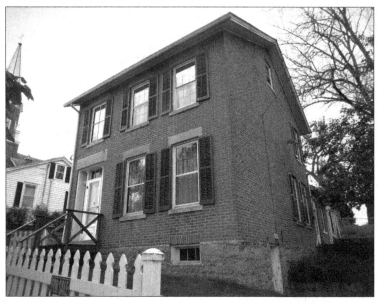

Grant's pre-Civil War home — 121 S. High Street

High Street

Grant's pre-Civil War Federal-style two-story red brick home sits high on a bluff above the Galena business district. It is the second house north of the Lutheran church near the corner of High Street and Washington Street, and it is here where Grant, his wife Julia, and four children lived. The house backs onto the old city cemetery and only cost them $100 a year to rent. His brother Simpson, the one ailing from tuberculosis, also moved in. (Simpson would later die from tuberculosis in September 1861.)

From this location, Grant could easily get to his job, church, and the rest of Galena by foot.

The houses on either side of the home were there when the Grants lived there. The Lutheran church, two doors south, was built in 1864 (three years after Grant left for the Civil War). With so many very pretty and historic houses on our entire route, no attempt will be made to describe them all. You'll see that many of them have been converted into small guest houses, bed and breakfasts, and the like. Any of them would probably be a fantastic place to stay for a quiet vacation.

But before heading toward the center of town, we'll turn left (north) and walk toward the corner of High and Hill Streets. Be sure to check out the yard of Grant's neighbor to the north. You'll see a totem pole, a dinosaur, and other imaginative decorations in the yard. I think that it is safe to say that the totem pole and dinosaur were not there when the Grants lived next door.

Hill Street

When we reach the corner of Hill and High Streets, we'll turn left to head west on Hill. You'll see a very interesting building almost immediately after making the turn at 408 Hill Street. It was built in 1855 as a German Methodist Church and is now housing. It's interesting to think that there were enough German-speaking Methodists in Galena in the 1850s to support their own church.

When you reach the next street (Dodge Street), keep heading west. The sidewalk will have two small sets of stairs. At 510 Hill Street, you'll reach a very well-kept and pretty 1840s-era brick Federal-style home. If you walk a little further west you'll see two cottage-like circa-1856 Italianate-style gable-front homes sitting side by side on the other side of the street.

The house on the right, 515 Hill Street, was the home of William Rowley, and house on the left, 517 Hill Street, was the home of John Rawlins. Both of them were close friends of Grant and both played important roles in his life.

Rowley was a clerk at the circuit court and met Grant when he installed some leather for a chair at the courthouse. During the Civil

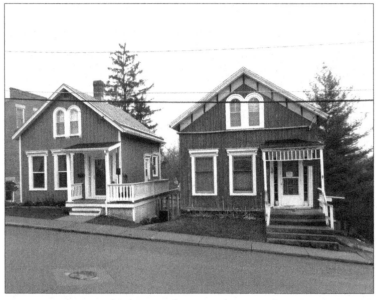

The homes of William Rowley and John Rawlins — 517 and 515 Hill Street

War, Rowley served on Grant's staff and was promoted to general at the end of his service. (Galena produced a total of nine generals during the Civil War.) After the war Rowley returned to the circuit court and eventually became a judge.

Rawlins was a local lawyer[3] and met Grant while doing some legal work for the Grant leather business. During the Civil War, Rawlins became a general and served on Grant's staff as his closest confidant, advisor, and right-hand man. More importantly, he took on the role of what we would now call a sober companion to make sure that Grant did not succumb to temptation to drink. Rawlins' efforts made sure that Grant kept his focus on the task at hand.

Grant was obviously ashamed of his weakness regarding alcohol and had this to say about Rawlins in his *Memoirs*. *"Rawlins remained*

3. My Great Grandmother's uncle, David Sheean, was John Rawlins law partner.

with me as long as he lived, and rose to the rank of brigadier-general and chief-of-staff to the General of the Army.... He was an able man, possessed of great firmness, and could say "no" so emphatically to a request.... General Rawlins was a very useful officer in other ways than this. I became very much attached to him."

When Grant became President in 1869, Rawlins served as Secretary of War until he died of tuberculosis a few months later. The only two faces on Galena's 1882 Civil War monument on the other side of the Galena River are of Grant and Rawlins.

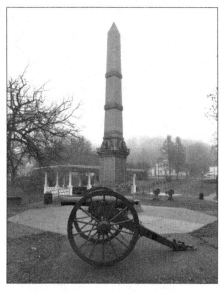

The Civil War Monument in Grant Park

Washington Street Steps

From here, we'll walk back to Dodge Street and then turn right (south) to follow the sidewalk to the corner of Dodge and Mars Streets (the next street). There is a very nice 1850s-era Federal-style red brick house at the corner. We'll cross the street to the sidewalk passing through Old Cemetery Park to Washington Street. The old cemetery is worth checking out if you're not walking with a dog. (Dogs are not allowed.)

At Washington Street we'll turn left (east) and walk pass the back entrance of St. Mathew's Lutheran Church to the corner of High and Washington Streets. Grant's pre-Civil War home is just off to the left (north). The house immediately to our left at the northwest corner of the intersection is from the 1850s. The house kitty-corner from

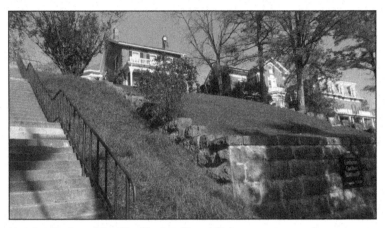

Nearing the top of the Washington Street Steps

us (the southeast corner) is from the 1840s. Both houses would have been here when Captain Grant walked these streets.

From here, we'll cross High Street to continue on Washington and then walk past the "No Outlet" sign to the sidewalk at the end of the street. For an explorer on foot, a "No Outlet" sign should be a signal to keep going. There is always the possibility that you might find a path or another way to continue your adventure. But you won't know for sure unless you check it out. In the case of Washington Street, we'll find a public stairway at the end of the sidewalk.

The house to our right at the top of the stairs was built about the same time that Grant lived in the neighborhood. The house to our left (Lamberson Guest House) was built after Grant's time in the neighborhood.

The Washington Street steps will take us down to the business district. In Grant's day the steps were made of wood. Today they are concrete. The stairs cross Prospect Street, Bench Street, and end at Main Street. It's 57 steps down to Prospect; 158 more steps down to Bench; and 37 more steps in the form of sidewalk steps down to Main; for a total of 252 steps.

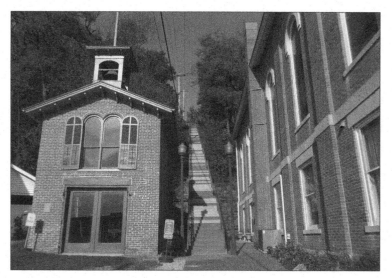

Middle portion of the Washington Street Steps

Bench Street

Before going all the way down to Main, we'll stop at Bench Street. The old 1851 Firehouse # 1 will be on our right. Take a look through the window and you'll see a vintage firefighting vehicle. The two-story house south of the firehouse (the one with the four posts in front of it) dates from 1838.

The "Galena and U.S. Grant Museum" is two more houses to the south at 211 S. Bench. The museum charges an admission and has many exhibits on the Civil War, Grant, and Galena including a replica of the Grant leather store. One of the exhibits is a huge painting by the famous 19th-century cartoonist Thomas Nast of Robert E. Lee surrendering to Ulysses S. Grant called *Peace in the Union*. But the most interesting exhibit might be an actual lead mine that was found under the museum building. It is the only lead mine in Galena that you can still see. The other lead mines in Galena have all been covered and remediated.

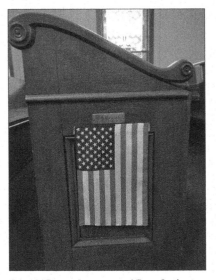

Grant's Pew – Courtesy of Rev. Catiana McKay

Immediately to the left (north) on Bench Street at the bottom of the stairs is the 1857 First United Methodist Church at 125 S. Bench. This is where the Grant family attended church services. You can even go inside and sit in the Grant family pew. (The pew is identified with a small plaque and an American flag.) Check at the door of the church to see if there is anyone inside who can let you in.

Before leaving the church area, you might want look underneath the lower part of the Washington Street Steps. There you'll see where the church has built a quiet place to sit. If you're looking for a place to meditate, this may be it.

If you walk a third of a mile north on Bench Street to the corner of Bench and Meeker Streets you'll reach the Jo Daviess County courthouse. Meeker Street is one street north of Franklin Street. The courthouse has been remodeled more than once since Grant's day, but the courthouse is where a major turning point in Grant's life took place. The front of the courthouse that you see today was built in 1900. The stone structure behind the front building is the court-house of Grant's day. There are newer portions of the building behind the original courthouse. We'll revisit Grant's life-changing events at the courthouse after we visit the Grant leather store down on Main Street.

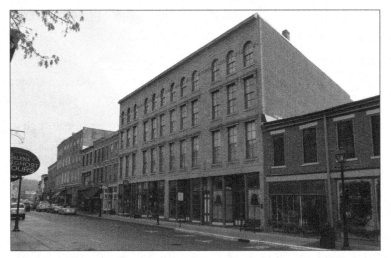

The Coatsworth Building where the Grant leather business was located

Main Street

To reach the store, we'll take the 37 sidewalk steps along Washington Street down to Main Street. This portion of Washington Street is a truncated red brick road no longer open to traffic. (It is open to delivery trucks.) You'll see a small pocket park at the base of the stairs with benches where you can take a break to get your bearings.

The location of the former Grant leather store is across the street from the pocket park and a bit to the left in the Coatsworth Building at 120-122 S. Main. (The leather store was at 122 S. Main.) The Coatsworth Building is the large four-story cream colored brick building that rises above its neighbors. The cream colored brick may have come from Milwaukee. (Milwaukee is famous for its 19th-century cream colored brick buildings.)

In the 1960s and 70s there were urban renewal proposals to modernize the business district by tearing down several buildings on Main Street, including the Coatsworth Building. The Coatsworth Building location was slated to become senior citizen housing. Had that happened, there is a good chance that you wouldn't be here right now following Grant's path. And certainly all the cars and pedestrians that you see on Main Street today would not be here. The essence of what attracts people to Galena today would have been thrown away.

Frank Einsweiler the mayor of Galena from 1973 to 1985 recognized that it was the concentration of 19th-century architecture that gave Galena its identity and fought the proposal. Ironically a few years earlier Jane Jacobs, the author of the classic book on what makes communities work, *The Death and Life of Great American Cities*, was fighting similar forces in her part of the world to protect her neighborhood in New York City from urban renewal. Einsweiler did make a compromise regarding the Coatsworth Building. The Coatsworth Building was completely renovated to include senior citizen housing units on the top three floors of the building.

Getting back to Grant and his Galena, you can see how the Washington Street Steps provided a direct connection between the store and his home at the top of the bluff on High Street. Before continuing with our tour, it's worthwhile to take a brief break to discuss the Galena that Grant moved into just before the Civil War and the life-changing events that occurred for Grant at the courthouse.

Galena in 1860 and 1861

When Ulysses S. Grant moved to Galena in the spring of 1860, the country was torn apart by slavery. Positions ranged from advocating outright abolition of slavery or containing it to where it existed or allowing for the unlimited expansion of slavery into the new territories or allowing the new territories to decide on slavery for themselves. The issue fractured the nation into four political parties.

The Republican Party, which generally consisted of northerners from the former Whig Party, ranged in views from full abolition to containing slavery. The Republicans selected Abraham Lincoln of Illinois who wanted to contain slavery to where it existed as a compromise candidate.

The Democratic Party split in two. The southern Democrats who wanted no restrictions on the expansion of slavery and were willing to break up the Union to get their way selected Vice President John Breckenridge of Kentucky as their candidate. The northern Democrats selected Stephen A. Douglas of Illinois who wanted to let the territories decide on slavery for themselves as their candidate.

The fourth political party consisted conservatives and southerners from the former Whig Party. They called themselves the Constitutional Union Party and selected John Bell of Tennessee as their candidate. They wanted to preserve slavery without breaking up the union.

Ulysses S. Grant was also split apart. His wife, Julia, came from a slave-holding family in Missouri. His father was an ardent abolitionist. Grant tried to split the difference by generally supporting Stephen Douglas. It really didn't matter because Grant had not lived in Illinois long enough to be eligible to vote.

With a split opposition, Abraham Lincoln won the election in November 1860. Not willing to wait to see what would happen, seven Southern states (South Carolina, Georgia, Florida, Alabama, Mississippi, Louisiana, and Texas) seceded from the Union and started their own Confederacy before Lincoln was inaugurated in March 1861.

Three days after the Confederates fired on Fort Sumter in South Carolina on April 12, 1861, Lincoln called upon the remaining Union states to raise volunteers to put down the rebellion. With that, four more states (Virginia, North Carolina, Tennessee, and Arkansas) seceded and the Civil War was on.

Upon receiving word of Lincoln's request for volunteers, the citizens of Galena (like citizens of towns all across the North) held a town meeting at the Jo Daviess County Courthouse at the intersection of Bench and Meeker Streets. The meeting began with the town's Democratic mayor urging compromise with the South. The crowd, incensed by the firing on Fort Sumter, did not want to hear this. Galena's Republican Congressman and friend of Abraham Lincoln, Elihu Washburne, gave a speech rebutting the mayor. Grant's friend John Rawlins, who was a Democrat, gave a rousing 45-minute speech saying that time for compromise was over and that it was now time to fight.

Upon leaving the meeting, Grant's friend William Rowley said to him, *"It was a fine meeting after all."* To which Grant replied, *"Yes, we're about ready to do something now."* With that, Grant, now with a purpose, was fully committed to the Union cause and never set foot in his father's leather store again!

Because of his military experience, Grant was asked to preside over a follow-up meeting held in the courthouse two days later to start the process of assembling volunteers for the upcoming war. It was during this time that Grant became further acquainted with Congressman Elihu Washburne who played a significant role in advancing his career.

Local volunteers wanted Grant to be their captain, but he declined as he believed that his background warranted a higher position with more responsibility. He did agree to drill and advise the local units. Grant accompanied the volunteers when they went to the state capital of Springfield on April 25 and stayed with them until they were assigned to a regiment. Grant remained in Springfield to help where he could while waiting for a suitable position to present itself.

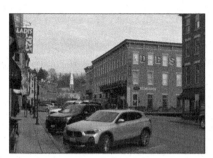

The DeSoto House Hotel

Continuing with Our Tour of Grant's Galena

Before getting ahead of ourselves regarding Ulysses S. Grant, we should resume our tour of Grant's Galena by heading south from the pocket park at the foot of the Washington Street Steps. We'll proceed on Main Street and walk toward the next street – Green Street. Although the stores on Main Street are clearly from the 21st century and generally cater to visitors, many of the buildings housing the stores were standing when Grant walked down this street. Most of the buildings in Galena have a metal marker identifying when the building was built along with a brief history of the building.

The 1853 DeSoto House Hotel at the northeast corner of Green and Main Streets is where Grant had his 1868 and 1872 Presidential Campaign Headquarters and where Abraham Lincoln gave a speech from the hotel balcony in 1856. Today's three-story building had two additional stories during Grant's time. The top two stories were removed in 1880.

Crossing the Galena River

At Green Street we'll turn left and head east toward the levee. There are public restrooms at the Galena City Hall just before we reach the levee. During Grant's time the area of today's levee was an active port and industrial area. Today's levee and the flood gates further down Main Street were completed in 1951 for flood protection.

When we reach the levee, we'll take the steps (32 steps) up to the top of the levee. The levee has a great walking path along the top, but for our walk we'll take the pedestrian bridge over the Galena River to Grant Park. Don't hesitate to turn around and take in the fabulous views of the Galena skyline as you cross the river. Can you imagine what the river must have been like when it was wider, deeper, and full of river boats and barges? Somewhere down there is where the Grant family debarked from the *Itasca* to restart their life in Galena.

Once we cross the river, we'll pass over the Galena River Trail and the Canadian National Railway tracks before dropping down into Grant Park. The Galena River Trail was once a Burlington Route (a predecessor to the BNSF Railway) branch line connecting Galena to the Burlington mainline running along the east bank of the Mississippi River. The Canadian National track is the original Illinois Central rail line coming into Galena from Freeport and points east and south in 1854. By 1855 the Illinois Central made it to the Mississippi River at Dunleith (today's East Dubuque). The railroad finally completed a bridge over the Mississippi River in 1869 to enter Dubuque, Iowa.

Grant Park

Our route follows the sidewalk at the end of the pedestrian bridge through Grant Park to Park Avenue across from Van Buren Street. Along the way we'll pass the 1891 U.S. Grant statue and the park gazebo. The 1882 Civil War soldiers monument with the sculptured

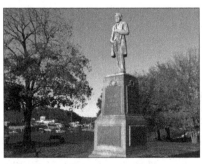

faces of Grant and Rawlins is on the north side of the park.

From here we'll cross Park Avenue and continue east on the Van Buren Street sidewalk to the steps at the end of the street. The steps lead up to Grant's post-Civil War home. The house next to the

Grant Statue in Grant Park

sidewalk and fronting on Park Avenue was built in the 1880s. Grant's last visit to Galena was in 1883.

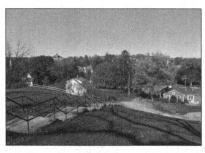

Van Buren Street Steps

Van Buren Street Steps

The Van Buren Street Steps has three sections. The first section of 40 steps goes up to a sidewalk; the sidewalk with 5 more steps leads to a driveway (actually part of 3rd Street); once you cross the driveway, the final section of stairway with 60 steps leads to a huge green lawn in front of the Grant house. The 105-step route was built by the city to make it easier for visitors to walk from downtown to the Grant house. The red brick path from the top of the steps to the house passes a statue of Julia Dent Grant. The statue was unveiled in 2006.

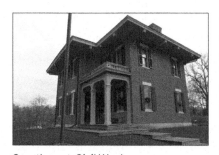

Grant's post-Civil War home

Grant House

The Italianate-style Grant house was built in 1859 and presented to the Grant family by several prominent Galena Republicans in 1865 as a thank you for his services during the War. Since Grant was still in charge of the Army and had responsibilities in Washington, Grant did not live in the house full-time. He did use the house as his residence when he ran for President in 1868 and 1872. The house is now owned by the State of Illinois and is open for tours.

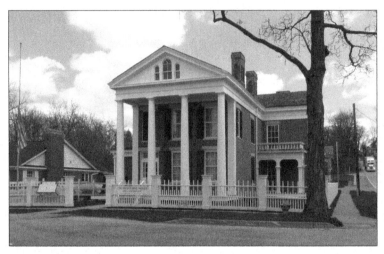

Elihu Washburne house

Elihu Washburne House

From the Grant house we'll take the short stairway down to Bouthillier Street (Grant's house faces Bouthillier), cross the street, and walk west on the red brick sidewalk on the other side of the street. Very soon, there will be a wide mulch path going off to the left. You may not notice the path if there are a lot of leaves on the ground. But if you've gone beyond the red brick sidewalk and are now on a concrete sidewalk, you've gone too far.

The path is actually an extension of 4th Street. Because of Galena's broken topography many of the city's streets were platted but never built. This type of street is known as a "paper street," as it exists only on paper. If you are an explorer by nature, you might want to check out some "paper streets" where you live. They might make for an interesting walk.

We'll turn left (south) at the path. The limestone house facing Bouthillier Street just beyond the path was built around 1840. While on the path, we'll pass an 1830s-era house in need of serious repair.

When the path reaches 4th Street, there will be a red concrete side-walk on the right. Just follow the sidewalk as it turns right (west) at Decatur Street (U.S. Highway 20) to the 1844 Greek Revival house of Congressman Elihu Washburne House at the corner of 3rd Street and Decatur.[4]

Elihu Washburne, who we met earlier when we were discussing the April 1861 courthouse meetings, was instrumental in advancing Grant's career. When Grant accompanied the Galena volunteers to Springfield, Washburne put in a word to the state governor on Grant's behalf. After performing various duties to help organize the army in Illinois and then going through some run around, Grant was finally appointed colonel of the 21st Illinois regiment in June 1861.

With the rapid expansion of the Union army, Lincoln asked Congress to submit nominations of qualified candidates to become generals. Again Washburne was there to offer Grant as a nominee. With that, Grant was promoted to general in August 1861. Grant continued to be promoted as he achieved success on the battlefield. When Grant had setbacks, Washburne was there to defend Grant from his critics. By the end of 1863, Grant was placed in charge of the entire Union army. He went on to win the Civil War in 1865 and was inaugurated President in 1869.

Had Grant remained in Missouri and not made the acquaintance of Elihu Washburne, there is no way that he would have had the career that he had! And what a Horatio Alger story it is to go from the depths of despair at the beginning of 1860 to President of the United States nine years later.

The Elihu Washburne house played other roles in Grant's life. When Grant was drilling the Galena volunteers in April 1861, it is

---

4. My Great Grandmother's father, Thomas J. Sheean (a Galena attorney), bought the house from the Washburne family in 1882. My Great Grandmother lived in the house during her teenage years and had her wedding reception in the house.

believed that they drilled on Elihu Washburne's lawn. In 1861, the property to the north of the Washburne house was vacant and part of the lawn.

When Grant ran for President in 1868 and 1872, he went to Wasburne's house on election night to receive the returns. (Wasburne's parlor was equipped with telegraph service for receiving the returns.) And it was in Elihu Washburne's parlor that Grant learned that he had been elected President of the United States.

Elihu Washburne served in the Grant administration as Minister to France. He was in France during the Franco-Prussian War of 1870-71. Grant and Washburne had a falling out when Grant sought the nomination of the Republican Party for a third term as President in 1880. (He had been out of office for four years and hoped to return.) With a deadlocked convention, James A. Garfield became the eventual nominee. Grant believed that Washburne had a role in his not getting the nomination.

The Elihu Washburne House is now owned by the State of Illinois and is occasionally open for tours.

Finishing Up Our Tour of Grant's Galena

To continue on with our Grant's Galena walking tour, we'll continue north on 3rd Street (going away from the Washburne house). At the end of the street we'll find a small wooden stairway with 30 steps leading down to a small playground park. We'll walk across the park lawn back to Bouthillier Street and turn left (west).

When you get near the intersection of Bouthillier and Park Avenue, you'll see the ornate red brick Italianate-style Waterworks building on the other side of the street. It was built after the Grant era in 1886. At the end of Bouthillier you'll find the 1857 Illinois Central Railroad station. This was Galena's train station when Grant and the

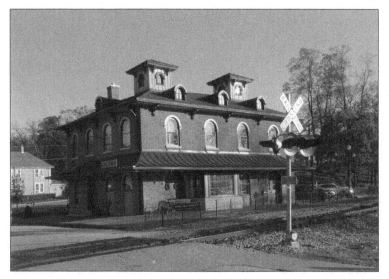

1857 train station

Galena volunteers left Galena for Springfield by train in April 1861 to join the Civil War.

This is a good place to conclude our tour of Grant's Galena. From here, it is a short walk back to Grant Park and the pedestrian bridge back to the town center. An alternative is to walk through the parking lot south of the train station toward the continuation of the Galena River Trail just beyond U.S. Highway 20. There is 36-step stairway up to the highway bridge and the protected pedestrian walkway to the other side of the river.

The U.S. Highway 20 Bridge is named for the mayor, Frank Einsweiler, who saved Galena from urban renewal. Walking across the bridge and then continuing up Main Street is good way to see all that Einsweiler saved for us to enjoy today.

Main Street and the areas near it are covered in the next chapter (Chapter 3). In the meantime feel free to explore as many streets as you want in Galena. They are all interesting.

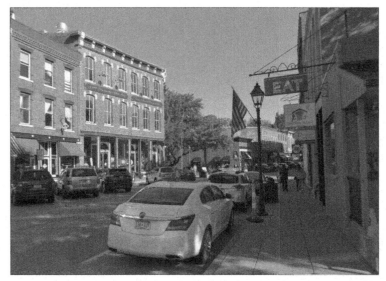

The view along Main Street from south of Washington Street

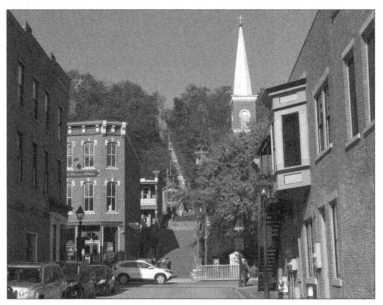

Washington Street and its steps

Chapter Three

A Tour Through the Heart of Galena

This walk through the heart of Galena begins where the walk in Chapter Two ended on the Frank Einsweiler Bridge over the Galena River. The walk takes advantage of Galena's public stairways to explore areas above and below the bluffs. This walk can be treated as one continuous walk or as a series of shorter walks. By the time you finish this chapter you will have covered almost all of what Galena has to offer.

This tour through heart of Galena begins on the west side of the Frank Einsweiler Bridge at the intersection of Spring and Main Streets and includes many of Galena's public stairways to explore Galena's central core and the historic areas that surround it. With Galena's steep hills, bluffs, and broken topography, public stairways are a convenient way to get from the bottom of a bluff to the top. A short stair walk can oftentimes eliminate a car ride of a mile or more.

Stairs also play an important role in Galena for relieving traffic on Main Street. Because parking can be tight on Main Street, visitors can park their car on Bench Street and then take steps down to the shops on Main. Because of this, the city has built new stairways to make it easier for visitors to get around.

Rather than a walk with a specific route, this walking tour describes the stairways starting from the intersection of Spring and Main Streets on the south and works its way north. (U.S. Highway 20 is called Spring Street west of the river and Decatur Street east of the river.) The stairway descriptions provide options for extending your walk and identify several places along the way to check out. The descriptions also include ways to connect to other stairways for a longer walk.

With more than 1000 historic buildings within Galena's heart, no attempt will be made to identify every historic building. The good news is that the presence of all these well-kept and very pretty buildings will make any and every walk you take in Galena a peaceful and wonderful experience.

As we begin walking north on Main Street, we'll see a paved pedestrian/bicycle path on our right-hand side near the river heading south and tunneling under Spring Street. (There is an interesting mural of a river scene inside the tunnel.) We'll continue north to the small park below the Galena Public Library on the west side of Main Street.

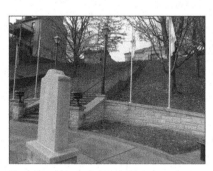

Veterans Memorial Park Steps

Veterans Memorial Park Steps (Main Street to Bench Street and then onto to the Library)

This small park honoring the town's veterans has several monuments, a bench, and a very nice and wide stairway with 61 steps heading up to Bench Street. The stairway has a nice approach at the bottom with urns and old-fashion street lights on either side. The Galena Public Library on the other side of Bench Street was built in 1907 and partially funded by Andrew Carnegie. There are 24 more steps on the other side of Bench to reach the front door of the library for a total climb of 85 steps from Main Street.

You can easily extend your walk by following the sidewalks on either side of the library to the backside of the library and then on to the Magazine Street Steps.

Magazine Street Steps (Magazine Street to Prospect Street)

The Magazine Street Steps can be reached from the library, or by starting from Spring Street and walking north to the junction of Main and Bench Streets. (This junction is before you reach the Veterans Steps.) From there, cross Main and follow Bench uphill.

The first street joining Bench from the left will be Magazine Street. Follow Magazine past the "No Outlet" sign. The steps are straight ahead at the end of the street. A pedestrian walkway ramping down to Spring Street will be to our left. (This walkway is another example of a "paper street" that has been turned into a pedestrian passage.) The backside of the public library will be on our right. (The Veterans Steps going from Main Street to the library can be combined with the Magazine Steps for a longer stair walk.)

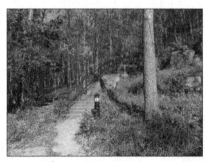

Magazine Street Steps

The Magazine Street Steps has 78 steps. The stairway has a railing on the left and very attractive waist-high light standards on the right. It climbs through a very pretty wooded bluff to Prospect Street at the top of the bluff.

At this point Prospect is a narrow private road open only to pedestrians and local residents and is a wooded wonderland. Right at the top of the stairs is Linmar Gardens. Linmar is the creation of local artist Harold Martin and, as can be expected, the gardens are very

41

imaginative. Linmar is privately owned and open to tours during the summer. (Contact Linmar Gardens directly to make a reservation.)

The gardens occupy 3 ½ acres on the side of the bluff. There are trails, steps, wonderful plants, water features, sculptures, a replica lead mine, and even the actual foundation of an 1844 African-American church. The entrance to the Linmar Gardens on Prospect Street has a very imaginative metal sculpture made out of an old heating oil tank.

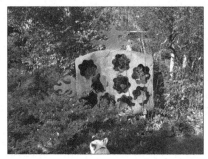

The Martinson sculpture

The metal sculpture is the creation of another local artist, John Martinson. If you are interested in seeing more of John Martinson's work, you can visit his West Side Sculpture Park at 620 S. West Street. It's only a few blocks away and doesn't have an admission charge. The park has an amazing collection of metal towers and other works made out of recycled materials that defy description.

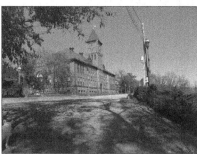

The old high school

If you continue walking on Prospect Street, you'll soon pop out of the woods just short of the old 1905 Galena High School building that dominates Galena's western skyline. The old high school is now a condominium development. The current high school is west of town on U.S. Highway 20. The Magazine Street Steps would have been major route for students walking to school when it was still a high school.

The views from Prospect Street looking down on Galena are fabulous. If you continue on Prospect you'll pass many wonderful homes one right after another. Many of the homes will be high above your shoulder and have stairways to reach their front door. If you are looking for a pleasant walk, continuing along Prospect Street is very hard to beat. You'll even find stairways at Green Street and Washington Street to take you back down to Main Street for a nice loop walk.

But for our tour and description of the Galena stairways, we'll return to Main Street to pick up our walk from the Veterans stairway below the library and head north. Almost immediately we'll run into the flood gates that protect downtown Galena from floods.

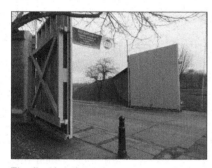

The flood gates

The Galena Levee and Flood Gates

The Galena River has a history of flooding and it still floods today. You can examine the outside of the flood gates to see how high the water has reached in past floods. There is even a sign to the right of the flood gates identifying the high water mark of a 2011 flood. Construction on the levee and flood gates began in 1949 and wrapped up in 1951 when the project was dedicated. A plaque commemorating the project is inside the flood gates on the west side of Main Street.

There is a very pleasant walking path with fantastic views of Galena on top of the levee. Three stairways provide access to the path. The one at the south end (24 steps) of the levee is just inside the flood gates; access from the center of town is at Green Street (32 Steps); and access at the north end (31 steps) is at the intersection of Water and Commerce Streets next to the old Blacksmith Shop. The north end has a monument noting the 2004 dedication of "The Pathway on the Levee Project." For those not wanting to climb stairs or are riding a bike, there is ramp access to the levee top at the north end.

Winery Parking Lot Steps (Main Street to Bench Street)

As you continue north on Main, the Galena Winery is a little beyond the flood gates on the left-hand side (west) of Main Street. At the north end of the adjacent parking lot there is a relatively new stairway of 54 steps connecting Main Street to Bench Street. This stairway was built to provide access to the shops on Main Street for people parking on Bench Street.

Warren Street Steps (Main Street to Bench Street)

There is another stairway with 46 steps that connects Main and Bench Streets a bit further north at the intersection of Main and Warren Streets. This stairway is much different than the others as it is narrower, made of wood, and has a fire escape landing on it near the bottom of the steps. And if you look to the south of the stairs, you can see that Warren Street is a grassy swale between Main and Bench Streets. The swale and stairway is another example of a "paper street" that is only open to those on foot. Like the Winery Parking Lot Steps, these steps make it convenient for someone parking on Bench to access the shops on Main.

From this point on, Main Street is a continuous string of shops and restaurants. No attempt will be made to identify them or to pick out favorites. All of the stores appear to be well-kept and seem to have plenty of foot traffic coming in and out.

Green Street – High School Steps (Main Street to Prospect Street)

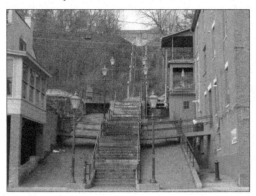

Green Street Steps

Our next stairway is at Green Street, one street north of Warren. The Desoto House Hotel at the northeast corner (on the other side of the street) is the major landmark for the intersection of Green and Main Streets. (See Chapter 2 for more information on the Desoto House.)

The Green Street Steps consists of an upper and lower stairway. The lower stairway has 43 steps connecting Main and Bench Streets and is built on top of a brick street now closed to traffic. It has metal railings and attractive old fashion street lights with metal posts. The upper stairway with 149 steps has very distinct concrete light posts with old style globe lights. It is set back from the west side of Bench Street and connects to Prospect Street high above on the bluff.

The sidewalk from Bench Street to the upper stairway passes in front of an impressive 1848 Italianate-style residence that is now a funeral parlor. At the south end of the funeral parlor's parking lot there is an arch-like brick structure built into the base of the bluff. It is all that remains of a root cellar for a house that used to be located there.

The upper stairway of the Green Street Steps is very pretty and has a very formal look with its distinctive lights. The stairway lands very close to the old high school and is also called the High School Steps.

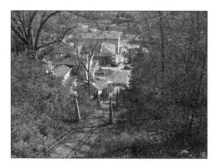
The steps from above

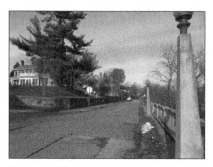
Prospect Street

There is a stone monument at the bottom of the upper stairway commemorating the restoration of the High School Steps in 1997.

Because of the 192 steps from Main Street to Prospect, one can easily save a half mile of driving to reach the top. With fantastic views at the top, the steps are a gateway for exploring the upper reaches of Galena. There you'll find very quiet streets with few pedestrians and wonderful well-kept old houses. A walk around these streets will make any trip to Galena special.

The High School Steps are also the site of the annual "Heroes for History Stair Challenge." The Challenge is held annually on a weekend close to September 11 as fundraiser for Galena's first responders and for the local historical society. It is a 5K race that involves running up the 149 steps of the High School Steps; turning right and running on Prospect to Hill Street; turning right again and running downhill on Hill Street to Bench; and then making yet another right turn to run on Bench Street back to the starting point to complete the loop. It takes seven loops (with a total of 1043 stairs) to make it a 5K race and to complete the Challenge!

The Green Street Steps are also a great link in a wonderful stairway loop walk. Take the stairs (192 steps up) to Prospect. Turn left and follow Prospect to the Magazine Street stairs (78 steps down). From the back of the library go around to the stairs in the front of the library (85 steps down) and take them down to Main Street. And complete the loop of 192 steps up and 163 steps down by following Main back to Green Street in the center of downtown.

Another great loop walk would be to turn right when you reach Prospect Street at the top and walk north to the Washington Street Steps and take those steps back down to Main Street. That option is 192 steps up and 193 steps down. You could even take the Washington Street Steps up to High Street and visit Ulysses S. Grant's pre-Civil War home (see Chapter 2 for details).

Washington Street Steps (Main Street to High Street)

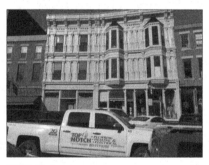

215 S. Main

As you continue north on Main Street from Green Street, you will pass an impossible-to-miss white building on the west side of the street at 215 S. Main. It was built in 1859 as a brick building. The sheet metal front was added early in the 20th century to give it a more "up-to-date" look.

Our next street and stairway is at Washington Street. This intersection has a small pocket park on the west side of Main Street. This is also where Main Street noticeably bends to the right. If it's a busy day, there is a good chance you'll see several people dressed in period clothes reenacting the Ulysses S. Grant era in the pocket park and maybe even see a musician or two sitting on one of the benches playing guitars. The Washington Street Steps begins here

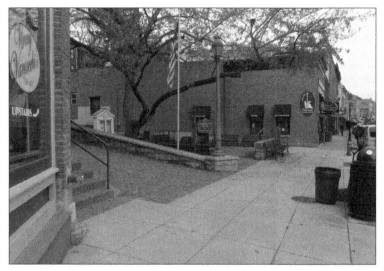

Pocket park at the base of Washington Street

and is prominently featured in the Ulysses S. Grant Galena Walk (Chapter 2).

With 252 steps from Main Street all the way to the top, the Washington Street Steps is the longest Galena stairway. The Steps consists of three sections. The lowest section with 37 steps is a sidewalk stairway on the left-hand side of a sloping narrow redbrick street that ramps up from Main Street to Bench Street.

The second section has 158 steps and is also called the Firehouse Steps. The steps are set back a bit from Bench Street and are wedged in between the 1851 Firehouse on the left (south) and the 1857 Methodist Church on the right. (This is where the Grant family attended church – see Chapter 2.) From here it is a straight shot up the side of the bluff to Prospect Street.

Once on Prospect, you have three options. If you turn left (south), you can continue on to the Green Street Steps or continue further south to the Magazine Street Steps. If you turn right, you can take

Prospect to Hill Street. There you will find another stairway going uphill from Prospect and a sidewalk with handrails sloping down to Bench Street and eventually down to Main Street.

But if you stay with the Washington Street Steps, you can climb the 57 steps of the third section of stairs up to the top of the bluff. When you reach the top, you'll have wonderful 19th-century homes on either side of you. The sidewalk at the end of the Washington Street steps will take you to High Street. Ulysses S. Grant's pre-Civil War home is off to the right at 121 S. High. It's the second house north of the Lutheran church (see Chapter 2.)

If you continue north on High Street to the next street (Hill Street) you'll pass more wonderful 19th-century homes and find a sidewalk stairway heading downhill on the north side of Hill. The sidewalk stairs end at an alley-like drive above Prospect Street. A more formal stairway on the other side of the drive completes the walk down to Prospect Street. From there you can loop back to the Washington Street Steps by going south on Prospect or Bench, or continue walking down Hill to Main Street.

If you continue west on Washington Street past High Street, you'll run into Old Cemetery Park. There is a pedestrian walkway cutting across the park to the cemetery and continuing on to the next street. The bottom line is that you have several great options for extending your walk.

We'll now return to the pocket park on Main Street at the bottom of the steps to continue our tour.

Hill Street Steps (Prospect Street to High Street)

Continuing north along the bend on Main Street, you'll see the next street is Hill Street. From Main, Hill Street is a steady ramp up to Prospect Street. The sidewalk from Main to Bench Street has hand rails for support on both sides of the street. The limestone building on the southwest corner of the intersection of Hill and Bench Streets is Galena's 1940s-era firehouse.

Next door to the firehouse to the south is Galena's Turner Hall (105 S. Bench). The building was originally built in 1874 and subsequently rebuilt after a fire and restored in more recent times. Today it is used as a civic auditorium and event center.

Several communities throughout the country that had a large number of German-American immigrants in the 19th century have (or had) Turner Hall buildings. Their origins come from an early 19th-century German movement to promote public health by establishing gymnastic clubs called Turnverein. The German immigrants built Turner Halls in communities where they settled as a combination of an athletic club, event center, and social gathering place. A prominent Turner Hall building is located in downtown Milwaukee, Wisconsin.

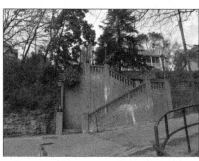
Hill Street Steps

Hill Street continues its upward slope to Prospect Street (the next street) after crossing Bench Street. At this point the hand railings are only on the north side of the street. At the end of Hill and on the other side of Prospect there is a very formal looking and impressive concrete stairway. It has old fashion black metal street lights and 59 steps to hop up the bluff. Because the face of the bluff is so steep here, the stairs go back and forth to gain height.

Once you reach the top of the formal stairs, you'll cross an alley-like drive and then proceed on a sidewalk with 33 more steps

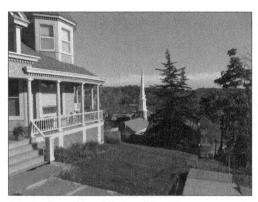

up to High Street (the next street) for a total of 92 steps between Prospect and High Streets. And once again, you'll pass impressive 19th-century homes and have wonderful views the entire way.

Hill Street sidewalk steps

When you reach High Street, you can turn left and walk to Washington Street and take the steps back to the center of town. Along the way, you'll pass Ulysses S. Grant's pre-Civil War home at 121 S. High.

If you turn right, you'll reach a pedestrian-only sidewalk passageway ramping down to St. Mary's Church on Franklin Street. The sidewalk has railings for extra support. You'll also see a small metal stairway on your right hopping up to Elk Street right where the pavement on High Street ends. As you walk down to the church you'll pass the now closed St. Mary's School. It is very dilapidated and is almost dissolving and falling apart right before your eyes. When you reach Franklin Street you can turn right and take the sidewalk back to Bench or Main Street.

Your third choice from Hill and High Streets is to continue straight ahead (west) on Hill Street to explore the streets above the bluff. The Ulysses S. Grant Galena Walk (Chapter 2) has more information on the area beyond High Street. Whatever direction you choose from the intersection of Hill and High Streets will end up being a very nice walk.

Perry Street (Main Street to Bench Street)

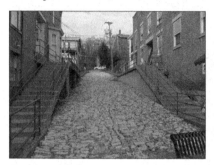

Perry Street

Perry Street between Main and Bench is a cobblestone street that is now closed to vehicles. The sidewalks on both sides of the street have steps (18 steps on the south/left-hand side and 19 steps on the north/right-hand side) with hand railings. The sidewalks continue as sloping ramps going upward after the steps.

Halfway up the south sidewalk there is a plaque on the wall adjacent to the sidewalk identifying it as the site of an 1832 stockade where early Galena settlers took refuge during the Black Hawk War. The Black Hawk War was a brief dispute between European-American settlers and Native Americans. Abraham Lincoln was captain of a volunteer company of the Illinois Militia during the Black Hawk War but never saw action.

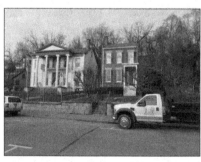

Bench Street houses

There are several fabulous houses at the top of the sidewalk where Perry Street ends at Bench Street. The white Greek Revival house with four large columns and the two green Liberty statues across the street and to the left at 120 N. Bench was built in 1840. The Liberty statues are a more recent addition. The Federal-style house just to the north of it at 122 N. Bench was built around 1850.

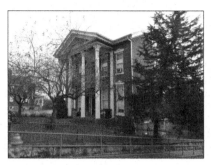

William Ryan house

Immediately on the north side of Perry adjacent to the sidewalk right where it reaches Bench is another Greek Revival house at 201 N. Bench. It was built in 1855 by William Ryan (a local businessman) who later moved to Dubuque.[1] His house in Dubuque, the Ryan House, is in Dubuque's Jackson Park Historic District (see Chapter 7).

The next stairway can be reached by making a right-hand turn on to Bench Street and proceeding north and across the next street (Franklin Street) to where Bench Street ends at Meeker Street. The next stairway is across the street and a bit to the left on Meeker.

Old Jail Steps (Meeker Street to Harrison Street)

The Old Jail Steps is the only stairway north of Franklin Street. The steps are across the street from the courthouse on Meeker Street and adjacent to the old jail that is now an inn. The courthouse was the site of a major turning point in Ulysses S. Grant's life. More information is in the Ulysses S. Grant Galena Walk (Chapter 2).

The Old Jail Steps has 88 steps and appears to be more remote and less used than the other stairways. But it is very interesting as it climbs into the woods to connect with Harrison Street up above. From the

---

1. William "Hog" Ryan was the brother of my Second Great Grandfather (James M. Ryan). They ran a wholesale grocery business and a meat packing business together in Galena. They dissolved their partnership in 1868, and William moved to Dubuque to open his own meat packing business and James remained in Galena to run his own meat packing business. James built the Ryan House a little over two miles west of downtown Galena on U.S. Highway 20 in 1876.

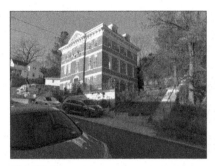

Old Jail Steps

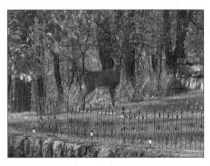

A Galena deer

top of the stairs Harrison begins as an unpaved lane through the woods that is now closed to vehicles. And it is a fantastic place to see deer!

Galena, like many towns, has an exploding deer population and a significant number of them live in this part of town. There are so many deer within the city now that the City of Galena has opened some isolated tracts of land to limited hunting. The bottom line is that it will be a rare day when you don't see deer on this particular stair walk.

Harrison Street remains lightly traveled when you reach pavement and you are still likely to see deer. For a nice loop walk, you can continue on Harrison and make a left-hand turn at Jackson Street (the next street). And then make another left when you reach High Street (also the next street). High will then curve to the left as it heads downhill to become Meeker Street. Be careful in the area of the curve as there is no sidewalk on this particular stretch of the road.

Perhaps, if enough people take this walk, a short path heading down to where High Street picks up again to the south can be cut through the woods right where the road starts to curve and High Street becomes Meeker Street. After all, the gap in High Street going through the woods is a "paper street" that is already owned by the city.

Since a path does not exist at this time, we'll remain on Meeker and will soon pass the old jail house where we started the climb. From here it an easy walk back to the center of town. If you continue walking east on Meeker, you'll soon cross a small creek and reach a pedestrian bridge over the Galena River at the end of Meeker.

Meeker Street Bridge and Galena River Trail

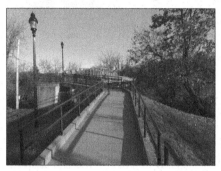

The Meeker Street bridge is at the end of Meeker. It is a pedestrian bridge over the Galena River and connects to the Galena River Trail on the other side of the river. The Galena River Trail is a rail trail on a now abandoned branch line of the Burlington Route. If you turn left on the trail and head north you'll reach the Buehler Preserve in around 1.7 miles. The preserve is a recreational open space next to the Galena River and is managed by the Jo Daviess Conservation Foundation. The preserve is open to hiking and has an ongoing prairie restoration project.

Meeker Street Bridge

The Jo Daviess Conservation Foundation manages and protects several other open space properties, including Casper Bluff, in Jo Daviess County. See Chapter 4 for more information on the Native-American mounds at Casper Bluff.

If you turn right after crossing the Meeker Street bridge, you can follow the Galena River Trail across from the center of Galena, past the old railroad depot, all the way to U.S. Highway 20. You will have fantastic views of Galena the entire way, and it is only about one half mile from the Meeker Street Bridge to U.S. Highway 20. There is

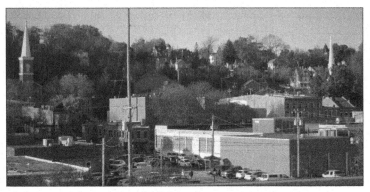
View from the Galena River Trail

a 36-step stairway up to the U.S. Highway 20 bridge to where we started our tour of the heart of Galena.

If you keep walking along the Galena River Trail, it will continue south of Galena all the way to the Mississippi River. You can even follow the trail to the base of Casper Bluff, where there is a steep trail up to the top of bluff. The top of the bluff has several Native-American mounds and fantastic views of the Mississippi River. The Galena River Trail ends a little over six miles south of the U.S. Highway 20 bridge.

Madison Street Steps

There is one more stairway in Galena that is now closed and no longer usable. It is at the intersection of Madison and Lafayette Streets on the east side of the Galena River. The 100 plus steps connect houses at the bottom of the bluff to what was once the First Ward School at the top of the bluff at the intersection of 4th and Madison Streets. The Italianate-style First Ward School building was built in 1891 and has wonderful landscaping. It has seen use as a residence and as an inn.

With this, our tour of the heart of Galena and Galena's public stairways is concluded. I'm sure you'll agree that Galena is fantastic place to take a walk.

Chapter Four

A Tour of East Dubuque's Dunleith Mounds

This walk through East Dubuque visits the best preserved Native-American mounds in the Galena–Dubuque area! Along the way we'll visit East Dubuque's Sinsinawa Avenue, catch a glimpse of the tunnel that made it possible for the Illinois Central Railroad to build a bridge over the Mississippi River to enter Dubuque, and get a spectacular view of the Mississippi River.

East Dubuque, Illinois (originally called Dunleith) for many years was known as an "open" city with late night closing bars, strip clubs, and gambling. East Dubuque's reputation as an open city began when Iowa adopted prohibition a couple of years before national prohibition kicked-in in 1920. East Dubuque retained its reputation after the repeal of prohibition in 1933 because Iowa still did not allow liquor by the drink. This meant that if you lived in Iowa and wanted a drink with your meal or to go to a bar, you had to cross the river to East Dubuque.

This all has changed as Iowa has had liquor by the drink for decades and the City of East Dubuque passed ordinances around a decade ago to shut down the strip clubs and to force the bars to close earlier.

But East Dubuque is more than its reputation. It has the best preserved Native-American mounds in the Galena–Dubuque area. And whether you come in from Dubuque or Galena, the East

Dubuque walk will begin by getting off U.S. Highway 20 at the east entrance of the mile-long plus Julien Dubuque Bridge over the Mississippi River and then heading north on Sinsinawa Avenue at the base of the bluff.

The avenue is named after Sinsinawa Mound a few miles away in Wisconsin. At 1,170 feet of elevation Sinsinawa Mound is the highest point in Grant County, Wisconsin and is the home of a Dominican Sisters community and retreat center. Depending upon the source, Sinsinawa means rattlesnake, home of young eagles, or clear water. All three names are applicable as the Mississippi River is right here; eagles do winter along the Mississippi; and rattlesnakes do live in the bluffs.

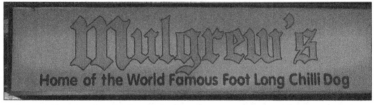

Sinsinawa Avenue is also East Dubuque's primary commercial strip and the one-time home to its famous strip clubs. With the strip clubs gone, finding a place to park on Sinsinawa Avenue is not difficult. Once out of the car, you'll want to walk north to where the avenue ends. Along the way you'll pass several bars. Although they no longer have strippers, they do have slot machines and many of them serve chili dogs. Mulgrew's at 240 Sinsinawa claims to be "Home of the World Famous Foot Long Hot Dog." So if you're hungry after your walk, you know where to get a chili dog.

When you reach the end of the avenue, you'll be at the junction of Sinsinawa and Jordan Avenue. Jordan is the red brick road heading up the drainage coming off the bluff. It is one of the most beat up roads that you'll ever find. It almost looks like it has been abandoned, and it could very well be closed to cars if there is a threat of snow or ice. This is where you'll turn to head up to the top of the bluff.

But before heading up Jordan, it's worthwhile to check out the railroad tracks of the BNSF and Canadian National Railways right at the end of Sinsinawa Avenue. If you like trains, you'll certainly see one if you wait long enough. The first railroad to reach East Dubuque (then called Dunleith) was built by the predecessor of the Canadian National, the Illinois Central, in 1855. This is the same rail line that passes through Galena. The Illinois Central reached Dubuque when it completed a bridge over the Mississippi River in 1869.

If you walk to the edge of the street, as close as you can get without entering railroad property, you'll see the portal of a railroad tunnel

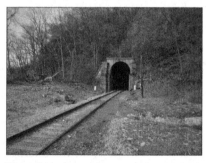

The railroad tunnel

punching into the bluff. The tunnel is the approach to the railroad bridge over the Mississippi. The railroad built the tunnel because there was not enough room in front of the bluff for a train to make the necessary turn the cross the river at a right angle. Instead the railroad makes the turn inside the 851 feet long tunnel. Once a train clears the tunnel, it has to cross the BNSF tracks at grade level before entering the bridge. The combination of the tunnel, turn, and grade crossing forces trains to slow down for the bridge crossing. This can sometimes cause a severe bottleneck for one or both of the railroads.

After checking out the tunnel, we'll head uphill on Jordan Avenue. With the red brick pavement being so beat up, you won't have to worry about cars whizzing by you. In fact, your chances of seeing a car on

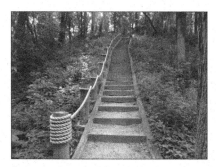

Steps to the mounds

Jordan Avenue are extremely small. Very soon into your walk you'll see a broad path with a wood beam and dirt stairway heading off to the right and going up to the top of the bluff. The path with 125 steps leads to the Dunleith Mounds in Gramercy Park.

The park and the nearby area is home to 26 Native-American burial mounds built during the Middle Woodland (or Hopewell Culture) period between 1500 to 2000 years ago. The Middle Woodland era (approximately 100 BCE to 500 CE) is when Native Americans began cultivating food to supplement hunting and gathering. This era is also characterized by pottery and riverside villages with conical burial mounds on nearby bluff tops. The Dunleith Mounds were investigated by archaeologists in the 19th century and in more recent times.

Without getting into too much detail but to provide some archaeological background. Native Americans entered North America during the Ice Age and hunted large animals such as mammoths and giant bison. This era is referred to as the Paleo-Indian phase. When the large animals became extinct, Native Americans relied upon a mixture of smaller game and gathering. This phase is referred to as the Archaic. The Archaic transitioned to the Woodland as agriculture and pottery were added to the mix.

Thanks to the efforts of the Gramercy Park Foundation, the mounds are well preserved and well kept up. If it were not for the Foundation, the mounds could easily become overgrown with trees and very difficult to visit. Instead, the lawn is trimmed so you can easily see the profile of the mounds, and there is a nice broad trail that

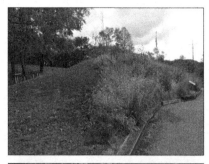

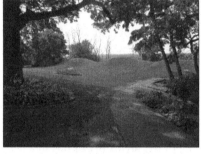

Some of the mounds

lets you weave in and around the mounds. One portion of the trail passes through a prairie grass restoration area. And along the way there are several comprehensive interpretive signs providing great background information on the mounds.

A visit to an archaeological site such as this is an opportunity to imagine what life was like when the mounds were built. At that time most of the land in the immediate vicinity would have been a prairie savannah with only a few trees. The bluff-top location would have been chosen for its dramatic view overlooking the Mississippi River. And the view today of the river and of Dubuque on the other side is still dramatic. The view alone is more than worth the walk to the top of the bluff.

Native Americans of 2000 years ago did not have horses, so any travel was by canoe or on foot. They would have used all of the land in the general vicinity to support a mixed economy of limited agriculture, gathering, hunting, and fishing. They may have even dug lead located near the surface to use for making paint and as a trade good.

Constructing the mounds would have been a community effort. Without modern metal tools, they would have used stone and wood implements to prepare the land and to dig soil for the mounds. Without wheel barrels, dirt to make the mound would have been carried to the mound site one basketful at a time. Based on the size of the mounds, it would have taken thousands of basketfuls of dirt to build a mound. The process of building the mounds must have been well-organized and probably included many ceremonies.

There is no doubt that there are many more mounds in the Galena–Dubuque area waiting to be discovered. (It wasn't until 1977 that the Little Maquoketa River Mounds – Chapter 9 – were discovered.) And one could make a serious hobby out of looking for mounds on the blufftops found all over the area. It wouldn't necessarily be easy as natural erosion has taken its toll to make many of the mounds unrecognizable. You would also need to obtain permission from a landowner to explore their bluff top. And finally you would have to develop the ability to recognize a mound sitting beneath the tangled undergrowth of a wooded bluff top. But an effort of this nature would have great value in adding to our understanding of the prehistory of the area.

Many of the mounds in the Galena–Dubuque area are from the Late Woodland era (500 CE to 1000 CE). The Late Woodland is when corn (maize) started to appear on the scene. The mounds of this era tend to be more linear and not as tall as the conical mounds in Gramercy Park. The Late Woodland era is also known for its effigy mounds in the shapes of various animals.

Examples of Late Woodland mounds including a "bird" effigy mound can be found at Casper Bluff Land & Water Reserve. The Reserve is about a five-mile drive south of Galena and is open to the public.[1] Casper Bluff can also be reach by bicycle by following the Galena River Trail south from Galena. The trail from the bike trail to

---

1. Driving instructions to Casper Bluff are as follows. From U.S. Highway 20 and 4th Street in Galena, turn south on 4th Street. It soon becomes Blackjack Road. Drive south 2.1 miles to the junction with Pilot Knob Road. Turn right on Pilot Knob and drive 2.4 miles to the Casper Bluff approach road. It is 0.4 miles to the parking lot where there is an information kiosk.

the top of the bluff is steep but very doable.

The grass above the mounds at Casper Bluff is not trimmed as regularly as the Dunleith mounds in Gramercy Park. As a result the Casper Bluff mounds may not be easy to recognize when you visit. (The mounds do have comprehensive signage to identify them.) The Jo Daviess Conservation Foundation that owns and manages Casper Bluff has reduced the amount of mowing it does to avoid soil compaction that could harm and possibly destroy the mounds. The Foundation has several other open space properties in Jo Daviess County that are open to the public for outdoor recreation.

There is another effigy mound very close to Galena at Keough Mound. Keough Mound is another Jo Daviess Conservation Foundation property. At the time of this writing, Keough Mound has been temporarily closed because of problems with sinkholes. The property will be reopened when the sinkholes are remediated. In the meantime, if you wish to visit other effigy mounds, Effigy Mounds National Monument in Iowa is only about 65 miles to the north.

Getting back to our walk in Gramercy Park in East Dubuque, you may have noticed a trail heading off to the right and downhill. That trail dips down into the side of bluff and then comes back up to the top of the bluff next to the picnic area on the other side of the park. The path has 69 stair steps.

When you are done exploring the mounds and checking out the view, you can return the same way you came up. You might even want to get a chili dog when you get back down to Sinsinawa Avenue.

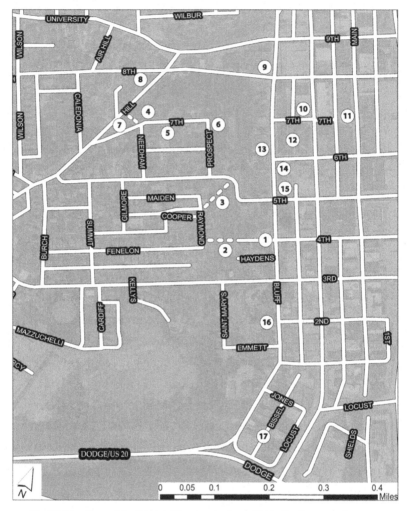

The Walking Tour of the Fenelon Place area begins at Cable Car Square at the intersection of 4th and Bluff Streets (Location 1). All location references are numbers in circles. Dotted lines are pedestrian passages.

1. Cable Car Square
2. Fenelon Place Elevator (Funicular/Incline Railroad)
3. 5th Street Steps
4. 583 West 7th Street
5. 548 West 7th Street
6. Paper Street (Prospect Street does not connect to 7th Street; it ends at the alley between 5th Street and 7th Street
7. Hill to 7th Street Steps
8. 8th Street Steps
9. Telegraph-Herald Building
10. Dubuque Museum of Art
11. Dubuque Town Clock
12. Washington Park
13. 605 Bluff Street
14. Historic Federal Building and Post Office
15. Redstone Inn
16. St. Raphael's Cathedral and Cathedral Square
17. Bissell Lane

Chapter Five

Wandering Around Dubuque's 4th Street – Fenelon Place Elevator Area

This tour takes in Dubuque's premier attraction (the Fenelon Place Elevator) and explores the wonderful areas that surround it. Along the way, you'll take in a couple of stairways, have some magnificent views, pass many great buildings, and run into a few surprises.

The 4th Street – Fenelon Place neighborhood west of downtown Dubuque is a great place to explore on foot. There is the funicular railroad at the end of 4th Street; fabulous 19th century buildings above and below the bluff; two very nice public stairways; wonderful views from the top of the bluff; Depression-era murals in the 1930s Post Office building; and many other surprises along the way. There is no wrong way to do this walk, and you are welcome to explore this area in any order you want. But for purposes of this narrative, we'll start at 4th and Bluff Streets (also called Cable Car Square).

Cable Car Square is a collection of predominantly 19th-century brick buildings with old fashioned street lights centered around the Fenelon Place Elevator (hence the name Cable Car Square) at the end of 4th Street. You'll also see that there are several little shops and places to eat surrounding you. For this particular narrative we'll be taking the Elevator up to the top of the bluff.

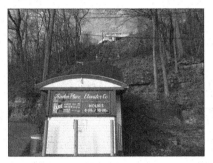

The Elevator from the bottom

This is a good place to check out the size and steepness of Dubuque's rugged bluffs to get an idea on how they have influenced Dubuque's urban landscape. You'll see that the bluffs are predominately limestone or other sedimentary rock. The only way for a road to reach the top is to follow a natural ramp provided by a drainage coming down from the top. The other choice for reaching the top is to meet it head on with a stairway or a funicular railroad as in the case of 4th Street. Before automobile usage became commonplace, Dubuque had many more stairways than it does today.

4th Street – Fenelon Place Elevator

If you are only passing through Dubuque and just have an hour or two available, the Fenelon Place Elevator is a must-do and must-see attraction. Especially if you like distinctive oddities that you're not likely to find elsewhere. The Elevator is open from April 1 to November 30.

The Fenelon Place Elevator is a funicular (or incline) railroad that climbs 189 feet along the side of the bluff from the end of 4th Street up to Fenelon Place. The original version of the Elevator goes back to 1882. The version that we see today with a few modifications goes back to 1893. The cable cars were rebuilt in 1977. The Elevator has been described as the world's shortest and steepest railroad, but this is difficult to prove as other funiculars have made the same claim.

A funicular railroad generally operates on the principle of two cars connected to each other by a cable and working together by counter-balancing each other. As one car goes downhill, it helps pull the

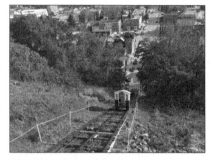

The Elevator from the top

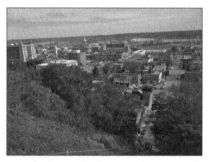

The view from the top of the Elevator

other one uphill. Because both cable cars are operating together at the same speed, the Fenelon Place Elevator only has three rails except in the middle where it bulges out to four rails to allow the cars to pass each other at the midpoint.

The motors that pull the cars and the operator who controls them are in the building at the top of the elevator. The top is also where you pay. You can board at the bottom and pay when you get off. The ride whether going up or going down is very cool and always has a bit of a bounce at the end. The view from the top is wonderful as you have a clear shot of downtown Dubuque, the Mississippi River, and the two bridges: one going over to Illinois and the other to Wisconsin. A ride on the elevator is great as a stand-alone adventure or as a wonderful way to begin or end an extended walking tour of this part of Dubuque.

When the Fenelon Place Elevator was built, it saved the 30 minutes or so that it took for a horse and buggy to descend from or climb up to the top of the bluff. Before the automobile changed all of that, funicular railroads were not uncommon in hilly cities. In fact, Dubuque had a second funicular railroad where the 11th Street Steps are now located (Chapter 6). Cincinnati, Ohio even had a funicular that carried streetcars from downtown Cincinnati up to the Mt. Adams neighborhood. You can also find funiculars in other countries.

If you get the urge to check out other funiculars (or inclines) after riding the Fenelon Place Elevator, you can travel to Johnstown, Pennsylvania; Pittsburgh; Chattanooga; or Los Angeles in this country. The Johnstown Incline was built after the devastating Johnstown Flood of 1889 to provide an escape route from future floods. Pittsburgh has two inclines on the banks of the Monongahela River across from downtown Pittsburgh. The Lookout Mountain Incline in Chattanooga is almost a mile long and goes to the top of Lookout Mountain. Angels Fight in downtown Los Angeles is about the same length as the Fenelon Place Elevator.

Continuing Your Walk from the Top of the Elevator

The first thing you'll notice from the top of the Elevator are the views. There are observation decks on both sides of the tracks to take them in. Assuming that you'll be exploring after your ride to the top, you'll pass a commemorative plaque describing the history of the Elevator on the outside of the Elevator entrance.

The street directly in front of the Elevator Building running north and south is Raymond Street. If you turn right on Raymond, you'll find the 5th Street Steps a couple of hundred feet to the north almost at the end of the street. If you're looking for a short loop walk, turning right is your best option. If you look left, you'll see Fenelon Place heading west away from the bluff. At one time there was a stairway heading down to 3rd Street at the junction of Raymond and Fenelon Place. Heading west on Fenelon Place offers several options for an extended walk.

Before going on an extended walk, we'll take a look at the 5th Street Steps.

5th Street Steps

The stairway at 5th Street has 127 steps and runs from 5th Street up through a park to Raymond Street. The stairway is in excellent repair and lighted. It is a very pleasant walk with many twists and turns as it works its way up the bluff.

If you're starting from Bluff Street at the bottom, follow the side-

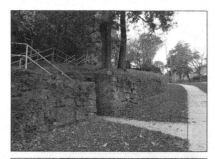

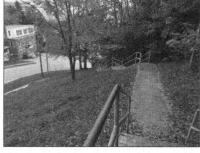

5th Street Steps

walk along 5th Street west from Bluff Street. 5th Street will turn to the right to gain some elevation. Just before 5th Street turns left to head west again, cross 5th to the sidewalk on the other side of the street. The stairway will be almost immediately to your left. It begins at the gap in the limestone retaining wall.

If you're starting at the top and going down, walk north on the sidewalk in front of the Elevator until it ends. The top of the stairway is at the far edge of the driveway of a relatively new residential development with the multiple gables, several garage doors, and a limestone front. Just think, if you lived here and worked down below in downtown, what a great walk you would have getting to work.

Heading West on Fenelon Place

Fenelon Place is a very pleasant street with a great mix of houses. Many of them are from the 19th century. As you head west on

Fenelon Place the first cross street that you'll reach is Summit Street. For our tour, we'll turn right and head north on Summit.

The Langworthy Historic District has several interesting homes and is less than a half mile west from here. The most unusual home in that historic district is an octagonal home built in 1857 at the corner of West 3rd Street and Alpine Street. The Langworthy Historic District is not part of this tour, but if you would like to check it out, you can turn left at Summit Street and head south to 3rd Street (the first street you'll reach). Then turn right at 3rd Street and head west to the historic district.

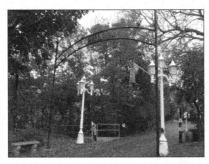

Steps to Hill Street up ahead

For our tour, we'll head north on Summit to where it ends at 5th Street. At 5th we'll turn right and head east to the first street where we can turn left (Needham Place) and then head north again. Needham Place ends at West 7th Street directly across from 583 West 7th Street.

You can't miss 583 West 7th Street as it has its address number mounted on a metal archway over the driveway with some very fancy old fashioned street lights along the drive. If you look closely at the driveway, you'll see that there is a stairway on the left-hand side just before the "No Trespassing" signs. The stairs are a public stairway going down to Hill Street. But before taking the stairs it's worth a few minutes to explore the area around West 7th Street.

If you head east toward the edge of the bluff you'll pass a house at 548 West 7th Street that looks like a replica of the White House. It's on the south side of the street. At the east end of West 7th there are two houses with incredible views. You can catch a glimpse of the

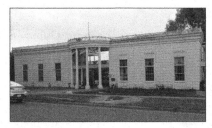

548 West 7th Street

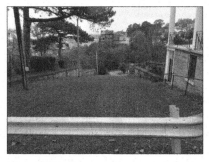

"Paper Street"

views by looking around the houses.

If you look to the south while you're at the end of the street, you'll see a stretch of grass sloping down to the street below. This is a good example of a "paper street;" that is, a designated street corridor that exists only on paper. At one time there was a public stairway along this street corridor. That stairway would have made it a much quicker trip to the base of the bluff.

After checking out West 7th Street, we'll return to the stairs and take them down to Hill Street.

Hill Street to 7th Street Steps

The stairway from Hill Street to 7th Street has 60 steps. The bottom of the stairway is at Hill Street where it begins as short sidewalk running perpendicular from the street. It soon turns into a stairway heading straight for the bluff. Once at the bluff it turns to the left and hugs the side of the retaining wall on its route up to 7th Street.

Our tour continues by turning right on Hill Street and heading northeast to 8th Street.

8th Street Steps

8th Street heading west from Hill Street is very unusual. The actual road is a steep uphill ramp supported by a retaining wall made out

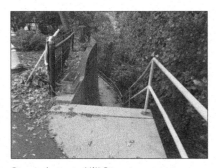

Steps down to Hill Street

of very large limestone blocks. As you walk around Dubuque you will become very familiar with very large limestone block retaining walls. They are everywhere and are ubiquitous to Dubuque. A typical retaining wall is usually made from very large blocks of Galena Limestone (or other hard forms of limestone). Each block must weigh tons.

The 8th Street sidewalk is more or less level and runs below

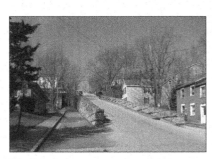

8th Street

the grade of the road as it proceeds west. At the end of the sidewalk there is a 35-step stairway to bring the sidewalk back up to the same grade level as the road. Both 8th Street and the sidewalk continue west as a steep route going uphill before leveling off. (Please note that the 8th Street steps were being repaired and were temporarily closed at the time of this writing.)

If you wish, you can continue west on 8th Street. There are many places where you can turn and start exploring. It is close to impossible to make a bad choice is this part of Dubuque; as it seems that every street has several interesting buildings and other worthwhile items to check out. You'll probably run into more retaining walls, steep sidewalks with steps, and very cool 19th-century homes.

But for this tour, we'll turn around and head east on 8th Street to

Bluff Street. 8th Street joins Hill Street and University Avenue in sharing a steep walled canyon that was carved by a natural drainage coming off the top of the bluff. The sidewalk along 8th Street is a good place to check out the geology of the bluff.

Telegraph-Herald Building

The Telegraph-Herald newspaper building is at the northwest corner of 8th and Bluff Streets and is wedged in between 9th and 8th Street

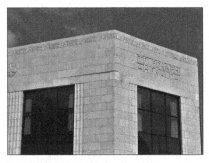

Telegraph-Herald building

at the mouth of the drainage coming off the bluff. In a city that has an amazing concentration of 19th-century architecture, the Telegraph-Herald building stands out as a classic example of late 1920s early 1930s Art Deco / Art Moderne architecture. It is a stone clad building with intricate designs carved into the stone. The name "Telegraph-Herald" is carved into the stone with an appropriate Art Deco font above the entrance at 8th and Bluff Streets.

The stonework, carvings, and the building's overall presence makes the Telegraph-Herald building a worthwhile and commanding stop on our tour. From here we'll turn south on Bluff Street.

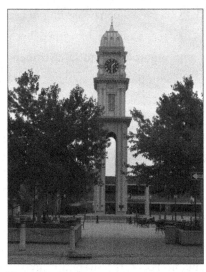

Town Clock

The predominantly 19th-century buildings on the west side of Bluff Street are tucked snug against the base of the bluff. As we continue south, we'll soon run into Washington Park, which occupies the entire block, on the east side of the street. The Dubuque Museum of Art is north of the park on 7th Street and well worth visiting. The Historic Federal Building and Post Office is south of the park on 6th Street. If you look east down 7th Street you'll see the Dubuque Town Clock and Dubuque County Courthouse with its gold dome. You are welcome to walk east to check out downtown Dubuque.

Just before reaching 6th Street we'll pass a massive red brick 1879 Second Empire-style building at 605 Bluff Street (on our right). The building was originally a single family residence that the Catholic

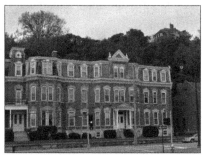

605 Bluff Street

Church converted into a safe boarding house for young single women working in Dubuque. With changing times and no longer a need for a women's boarding house the building has since been repurposed into an apartment complex.

From here we'll cross Bluff Street to check out the Historic Federal Building and Post Office on 6th Street.

Depression Era Mural Art

The Art Deco / Art Moderne-style Historic Federal Building was completed in 1934 and houses two Depression Era murals. During the Depression the WPA (Works Progress Administration) sponsored Post Office murals across the country to provide work for artists. But the murals in the Dubuque Post Office were not funded by the WPA; they were funded by the Treasury Department.

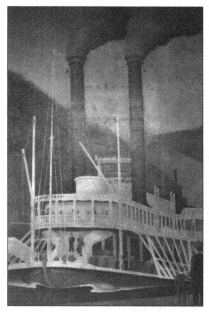

Early Mississippi River Packet (boat)
Dubuque III

When the mural competition was opened in 1934, the hope was to award the murals to Grant Wood of "American Gothic" fame. (Grant Wood grew up in nearby Cedar Rapids.) Wood declined to participate in the competition, and the murals were awarded to two of his students/associates. William E. L. Bunn painted "Early Mississippi Packet (boat) Dubuque III" and Bertrand Adams painted "Early Settlers of Dubuque." Both murals were completed in 1937 and are just inside of the central entryway on 6th Street.

The Historic Federal Building was acquired by the City of Dubuque in 2006 and was renovated and restored in 2007. The renovation included converting the courtroom into the Dubuque City Council chambers. The Post Office is still in the lobby and has a very dignified and impressive look with its walnut paneling.

Returning to Cable Car Square

After checking out the murals, we'll continue south on Bluff Street. At the very next street (5th Street) at the northeast corner there is a massive red stone house that is now the Redstone Inn. The Queen Anne-style house was built in 1894 by Augustin A. Cooper, who owned a wagon works, to give to his daughter as a wedding gift. After several incarnations the house is now an inn.

If you haven't climbed the 5th Street Steps, you can turn right on 5th Street and walk west to the stairway. From the top of the stairway, you can walk south to the Fenelon Place Elevator and take it back down to our starting point. Otherwise, we'll continue south on Bluff Street back to our starting point at Cable Car Square.

Extending the Walk to Bissell Lane

If you wish to extend your walk, you can continue south on Bluff Street. At 3rd Street you'll pass Cathedral Square and several buildings related to St. Raphael's Cathedral. St. Raphael's is the seat of the Archdiocese of Dubuque. Construction on the Gothic Revival-style cathedral began in 1857 and was completed in several phases during the 19th century.

Because of the large number of Irish and German settlers during the 19th century, Dubuque had and still has a very large Catholic presence. You'll see Catholic churches and other Catholic institutions everywhere. There are even two Catholic colleges, and in fact, Dubuque may be the smallest city in the country with its own Archdiocese.

After checking out the cathedral, you can keep going south on Bluff Street. After you pass 1st Street, you'll soon reach Jones Street. If you turn left on Jones and walk a short distance east, the next cross street will be Bissell Lane.

Bissell Lane is not much to speak of as it is much more of an alley than a lane. Almost all of what few buildings there are on Bissell Lane face other streets. But the lane does have some special significance as it is named for Richard Bissell.

Richard Bissell is not a name you hear very often today, but his 1953 novel *7 ½ Cents* was very popular at the time. The humorous novel is loosely based upon his experiences as a supervisor at his family's garment factory in Dubuque. The story is set in a pajama factory in a fictitious Iowa river city where the workers are asking for a 7 ½ cents per hour raise. Based upon a 40-hour workweek, that would have amounted to a $3.00 a week raise.

Bissell soon adapted the book into the award winning Broadway musical *The Pajama Game*. The most notable songs from the musical are *Hey There (you with the stars in your eyes)* and *Hernando's Hideaway*. Both Rosemary Clooney and Sammy Davis Jr. recorded *Hey There* for big hits in the 1950s. The musical was so successful that it was made into a movie of the same name staring Doris Day. The movie, too, was a big success.

With Bissell's huge success, the City of Dubuque wanted to honor him, and somehow the alley between Bluff and Locust Streets became Bissell Lane. Being a fan of the unusual and unwanted, Richard Bissell loved his namesake alley. And in a sense, finding and celebrating the quirky oddities along the way is what exploring on foot is all about. Since Bissell's day his namesake alley has had some truncation due to the transformation of the stretch of U.S. Highway 20 south of Bissell Lane into a multilane near expressway.

But there is enough of the lane remaining to give us a sense of its place in popular culture history. And with that our tour of the 4th Street – Fenelon Place Area of Dubuque is finished.

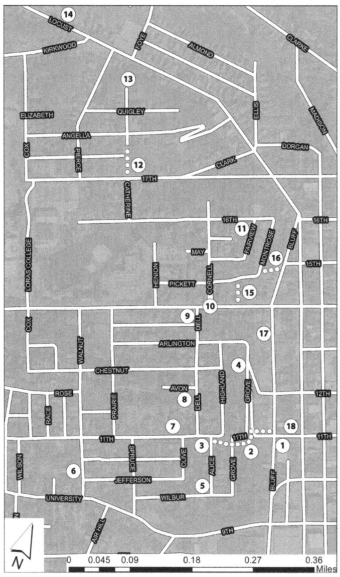

The Walking Tour of the West 11th Street area begins at the Carnegie-Stout Public Library at the corner of 11th and Bluff Streets (Location 1). All location references are numbers in circles. Dotted lines are pedestrian passages.

1. Carnegie-Stout Public Library
2. 11th Street Steps
3. 510 West 11th Street
4. 1207 Grove Terrace
5. Very Large Dubuque-Style Retaining Wall
6. 1025 Walnut Street
7. 563 West 11th Street
8. Avon Park
9. Mural on Building at Loras and Dell
10. Loras Boulevard Intersection with Two Cross Streets
11. 1595 Fairview Place
12. Paper Street with small stairway on Catherine Street
13. Unusable Stairway at the end of Catherine Street
14. Unusable Stairway on West Locust Street
15. Loras to Montrose Terrace Steps
16. Bluff to Montrose Terrace Steps
17. 1335-37 Bluff Street
18. Richardsonian Romanesque House

Chapter Six

Touring Dubuque's West 11th Street Historic District and Bluffs Nearby

This walk tours several of Dubuque's bluff top neighborhoods and passes many, many wonderful 19th-century homes. The walk also includes several stairways including one of the best stairways in the entire country! You'll also have plenty of chances to examine Dubuque's ubiquitous limestone retaining walls and will take in one Dubuque's many great murals.

This walk begins next to the circa-1901 Carnegie-Stout Public Library at the corner of 11th and Bluff Streets and heads west to explore Dubuque's West 11th Street Historic District. The Stout in Carnegie-Stout is for Frank D. Stout who donated the land for the library. Stout was a successful businessman and a mayor of Dubuque. His father, Henry L. Stout, amassed a huge fortune in the lumber business, and members of the Stout family built the large houses just

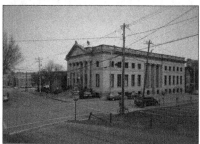

Carnegie-Stout Public Library

to the north of the library on Locust Street.

Before starting the walk, it's worth taking a few minutes to check out the inside of the library as it is quite grand. The historic district is on top of the bluff to our west. To get there we'll climb the 11th Street Steps. The steps begin as a sidewalk stairway kitty-corner from the library.

The West 11th Street Historic District is a fantastic area to explore on foot. The views are tremendous and every street has wonderful and distinctive homes. Many, if not most, of the homes are from the 19th century. The historic district itself covers the top of the bluff. It is bordered to the north by the Loras Boulevard corridor and on the south by the 9th Street and University Avenue corridor. Both corridors follow natural drainages that have carved ramps up to the higher ground west of the Mississippi River.

One hundred years ago, the Eleventh Street Elevator, a funicular railroad very similar to the Fenelon Place Elevator that we rode in Chapter 5, ran from right here (below the bluff) to the top. The portal in the retaining wall to the west was opened to accommodate the funicular. The funicular was shut down in 1927 and torn down in 1929.

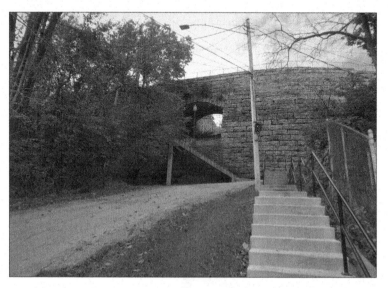

Bottom of the 11th Street Steps

As you begin walking west on the 11th Street Steps, you can't help but to notice the massive Dubuque-style retaining wall made out of enormous buff-colored limestone blocks right in front of you. As mentioned earlier in this book, retaining walls are ubiquitous to Dubuque, and you'll have plenty of chances to examine them on this walk. The other thing you'll notice right in front of you is the skyline of impressive homes above the retaining wall.

11th Street Steps

Walking up the 11th Street Steps is a fantastic experience, and as one who has climbed hundreds of public stairways in 19 different states and the District of Columbia, I can attest the 11th Street Steps is among the best. This stairway is almost magical. As already mentioned, the steps begins as a sidewalk stairway at 11th and Bluff Streets. Before reaching the retaining wall it becomes a stand-alone stairway held up by a concrete pillar and then passes through the portal

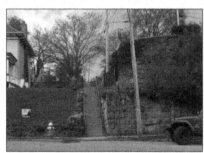

Steps continuing up to Alice Street

in the retaining wall. You'll be entering the historic district when you pass through the portal.

As you emerge on the other side of the portal and step onto Grove Terrace, it will almost be like Dorothy and Toto landing in Oz. It's as if he world has switched from black and white to full and living color. In every direction from left to right there are gorgeous and exceptionally well maintained Victorian-era houses. And with every house painted in a different vibrant color you'll find the historic district an incredible place to explore on foot.

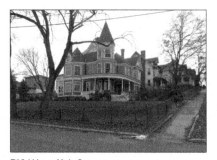

510 West 11th Street

But the stairway isn't done. It continues going up on the other side of Grove Terrace along the side of another large retaining wall to Alice Street. About a third of the way up from Grove, you'll pass a terrace off to the side of the stairway that features a place to sit, an overlook surrounded by an iron fence, and a commemorative plaque for the Eleventh Street Elevator.

When you reach Alice Street you'll see a very impressive circa-1895 Queen Anne-style home with a conical tower a bit higher up on the bluff on the other side of the street. It's on the southwest corner of 11th and Alice Streets at 510 West 11th Street. When you turn around, the view looking across Dubuque and the Mississippi is amazing. As for where to go next, you can't go wrong, and your best bet is to wander up and down as many streets as you have time for. You'll see impressive houses and have wonderful views on almost every street.

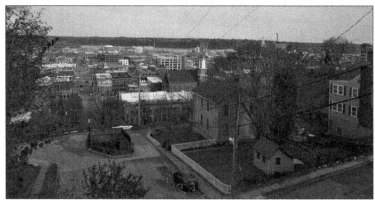

The view from the top

As for the number of stairs on the 11th Street Steps, the sidewalk stairway at the bottom has 37 steps. The middle section that goes through the portal and emerges at Grove Terrace has 72 steps. And the final section going up to Alice Street has 64 steps. That's a total of 173 steps (give or take a step or two for miscounting) from Bluff Street at the bottom to Alice Street at the top.

Exploring the West 11th Street Historic District

With so many wonderful options for exploring, it's hard to make a decision. So to drive a stake in the ground, we'll make a right-hand turn at the top of the stairs and follow 11th Street as it loops around onto Highland Place. The 11th Street Steps will be down below and to our right as we make the turn.

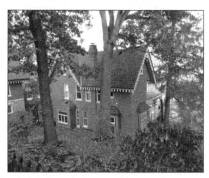

Backside of 1207 Grove Terrace

Highland will slope downward as we head north to Arlington Street. The houses on Highland will be to our left and a bit higher up the bluff. On our right and below us, we'll be able to see the backsides of the houses on Grove Terrace. Every house along way is worth a photo stop.

When Highland ends at Arlington Street, we'll turn right and continue downhill one more block to where it curves to the right and becomes Grove Terrace. There are amazing views of the city down below as we curve along the edge of the bluff.

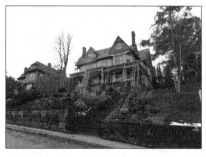

1203 Grove Terrace

As we walk along Grove Terrace the houses will now be on our right and above us. The edge of the bluff will be on our left. We'll still be trending downhill for a bit before sloping uphill. Again, all of the houses are fantastic on this street. Most of them are variations of Victorian-era Queen Anne-style houses. But keep an eye out for a ginger-bready wood trimmed circa-1856 Gothic Revival-style house at 1207 Grove Terrace. You won't be able to take your eyes off of it. All of the houses have great details, but 1207 Grove Terrace takes it up a notch or two.

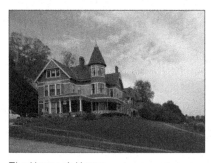

The Hancock House

In a short time we'll be back where the 11th Street Steps emerges from the portal. Grove Terrace will curve to the right and then to the left to get around the portal. As we follow the curve there is a very large Queen Anne-style home on our right called The Hancock House that is now a bed and breakfast.

Right now it's decision time. You can continue south on Grove Terrace or take the 11th Street Steps back up to Alice Street. If you continue south, Grove Terrace will end at Wilber Street. If you turn right (your only option) onto Wilber and then turn right again at Alice Street, you can loop back to the top of the 11th Street Steps.

The northwest corner of Alice and Wilber Streets has an enormous Dubuque-style retaining wall. This wall is quite interesting as it is a combination of natural bedrock and enormous limestone blocks. It provides support for a large house facing Olive Street up above.

If you're not ready to loop back to the top of the stairway, you can follow Wilber to where it ends at Spruce Street. Spruce Street is a

very steep street with handrails and several sidewalk steps thrown in
for good measure. If you turn right on Spruce you can take it uphill to
where it ends at 11th Street, and then take another right to bring you
back to the top of the 11th Street Steps.

Another option after turning right onto Spruce is to turn left at
the first street (Jefferson Street) and follow Jefferson Street west to
where it ends at the next street (Walnut Street). Immediately across
the street on the other side of Walnut is a short stairway going up to
what looks like to be a park. It's not. It is actually the broad lawn of

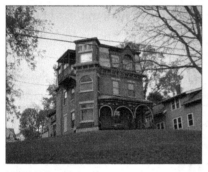

a very ornamental and eclectic
circa-1880 Queen Anne-style
house (1025 Walnut Street)
that has been converted into
a multi-family residence. In a
neighborhood that abounds
in houses that catch your
attention, 1025 Walnut, too,
is near the top of the list.

1025 Walnut Street

From 1025 Walnut, you can continue north on Walnut to 11th
Street. The house immediately to the north at 1051 Walnut, the
one with the wonderful landscaping, is a 1920s-era Craftsman-style
bungalow. The next house north is from the 19th century. When you
reach 11th Street you can turn right to return to the 11th Street Steps.
Before reaching Spruce Street, Prairie Street will head north perpen-
dicularly from 11th Street. Prairie Street, to no surprise, has its share
of 19th-century homes that you might want to investigate. When
you finally do reach Spruce Street, you'll see a frame house at the
southwest corner of 11th and Spruce that may go back to Dubuque's
lead mining days.

The Italianate-style house at 636 West 11th Street is believed to have been constructed in 1848. At that time, 170 plus years ago, the bluffs of Dubuque would have been loaded with lead mines. It would be fun to find a map showing where the old mines were located and to see if you could still find a mine opening. The best time to look for an old opening on the side of a bluff would be in the winter when there would be less foliage to obscure your view.

As for exploring more of the West 11th Street Historic District, every street has something worthwhile. There is no point in bogging down this narrative by describing every street. Your best bet is to wander where you want and to check out whatever catches your attention. But if you continue from 11th and Spruce back to 11th and Alice, you will see many great buildings along the way. One that caught my attention was a circa-1875 Second Empire-style brick house with a mansard roof and very intricate architectural details at 563 West 11th Street. It's on the north side of the street.

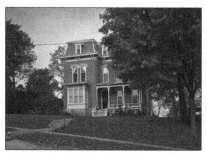

563 West 11th Street

Where to Go Next After Returning to 11th and Alice Streets?

With so many streets to explore in the historic district, you could stay right in this area to continue exploring. But there are two more public stairways on the northern edge of the historic district. One connects Loras Boulevard with Montrose Terrace and the other connects Montrose Terrace with Bluff Street.

The most direct connection from the top of the 11th Street Steps to the other two stairways is to head west on 11th Street for a few feet to Dell Street. Dell begins on the north side of 11th Street and looks

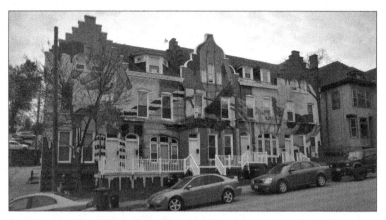

Amazing mural at Dell and Loras!

like an alley. Dell is for all practical purposes is the alley for Highland Place, but it does offer a straight shot down to Loras Boulevard. Dell Street becomes very steep at the very end as it descends into the Loras Boulevard corridor. You are welcome to vary your route.

A couple of hundred feet after making the turn onto Dell, you'll run into a very cool little playground park (Avon Park) on the west side of the street. The park is tucked into an almost secret location surrounded by other properties and is a good place to stop if you're ready for a break. Being more of an alley than a street, you'll see the back sides of many houses as you walk along Dell.

You'll cross Chestnut and Arlington Streets on the way to Loras. Just before reaching Loras, you'll see a limestone retaining wall with an iron fence above it on the west side of the street. If you look closely you'll also see a very tiny stairway with 13 steps going down to the roadway behind the buildings fronting Loras. Dell ends at Loras. At this point, you'll want to cross Loras and then turn right to head east. But before leaving Dell, make sure you turn around and check out the building facing Loras at the southwest corner of Loras and Dell.

The building is a circa-1895 Queen Anne/Dutch Colonial-hybrid multi-family residence with its entire front covered with a mural.

The multi-color mural is extraordinarily unusual as it features fingers caressing the windows, flower blossoms, and eagles soaring across the face of the building. It is definitely worth checking out. Colorful murals are a relatively recent addition to Dubuque's streetscape and are always worth a stop to check out. As you walk along Dubuque's busier historic streets, you might want to turn around every now and then to make sure you haven't missed a mural. You'll find them in the most amazing locations.

We'll continue our walk along the north side of Loras and head east. And without surprise there will be several great buildings with great details along the way for us to check out. Almost immediately after crossing Loras, we'll reach an intersection with two separate streets for us to cross. Just before crossing the two streets there is a very interesting house at 509 West Loras. It is a circa-1896 Queen Anne/Romanesque-style building with great windows in the conical third floor tower.

The Loras Boulevard Intersection with Two Separate Streets to Cross

The intersection with two cross streets on Loras is very interesting and worth taking some time to examine and explore. With Dubuque's hilly topography, residential streets are sometimes stacked up like the tiers of a wedding cake with each tier being set back from the one below it. In the case of this intersection, the near cross street, Cornell Street, is ramping up to an upper tier that is defined by 15th Street on the south and Fairview Place on the east. The far cross street, Montrose Terrace, proceeds to a lower tier defined by Montrose Terrace on both the south and on the east. Montrose at this point is at the same level as Loras at the intersection. But with Loras continuing downhill, Montrose Terrace will soon become a tier well above Loras.

If you follow Cornell uphill, you'll notice that Cornell and Montrose are separated by a Dubuque-style retaining wall. If you look closely at the wall, you can see where there were probably steps going down to Montrose some time ago. If you keep going uphill on Cornell to 15th Street and turn right on 15th, you'll see where 15th becomes almost as narrow as a sidewalk before reaching Fairview Place. As you walk north along Fairview, you will see stairways on the east side of the street leading down to the houses below. At one time, one or

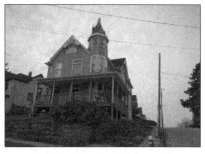

more of those stairways may have provided a connection to Montrose Terrace.

Fairview ends at 16th Street. At the southwest corner of the intersection at 1595 Fairview Place there is a recently renovated and

1595 Fairview Place

very cool house with amazing details. At this point you can turn east and walk to Montrose Terrace or turn west and walk back to Cornell. If you're a true stairway aficionado you may want to continue west on 16th Street beyond Cornell to check out two stairways that are no longer usable; otherwise, turn left on Cornell to return to the Loras intersection.

Checking Out the Two Unusable Stairways

The two unusable stairways are in the West Locust Street corridor. At one time when people got around on foot or relied upon transit, the stairways were an easy way for people living on top of the bluffs to get down to a school or a transit stop on West Locust Street. To visit the two stairways we'll continue downhill on 16th Street to Catherine Street (the next intersection). When we reach the bottom of the hill, we'll be at the eastern edge of the Loras College campus.

If you're looking for some more stairs to climb, there are stairways on the campus.

For our tour we'll turn right and head north on Catherine. Catherine will become a paper street after the next cross street (17th Street). We'll walk on the sidewalk that would have been the west side of Catherine Street. There is a very small 11-step stairway at the end of the sidewalk going up to the continuation of Catherine Street. Just keep walking north on Catherine past Angella and Quigley Streets. (These are both very short blocks.) The old 100-step or so stairway down to West Locust is at the end of Catherine (just past Quigley). The steps are closed and absolutely unusable. They are a twisted mess of concrete that the city will probably remove some day.

To reach the second unusable stairway, we'll have to backtrack a bit to Quigley and make right-hand turn downhill to Pierce Street. Turn right at Pierce and continue downhill to West Locust. At West Locust, we'll cross the street, turn left, and continue west past the old school building and its parking lot on the west side of the school. Right after you pass the parking lot, there will be a sidewalk heading north towards the bluff. There will also be a sign saying steps closed. At the end of the sidewalk there is another 100-step plus stairway going up to Hodgden Street. Like the stairway at the end of Catherine, this stairway is absolutely unusable and a total mess. It, too, will probably be removed by the city someday.

With that, our excursion to the pair of unusable steps is complete. It's now time to find our way back to Loras and Cornell where we will find two very nice and very usable stairways.

Loras Boulevard to Montrose Terrace Steps

After returning to Loras, we'll cross both streets of the intersection and continue east. Keep an eye out to the left because in a couple of hundred feet there will be a sidewalk wedged in between 465 and

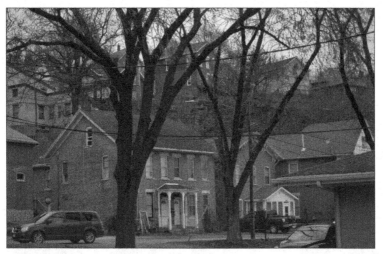

Tiers of houses

459 Loras Boulevard leading to a 28-step stairway up to Montrose Terrace. When you reach Montrose, you will have left the official West 11th Street Historic District. Our next stairway will be a short walk to the right.

Even though the tiers above Loras are not in the official historic district, they are, as we saw when we followed Cornell, well worth exploring. In fact, almost any Dubuque street that was developed before automobiles became commonplace is worth exploring on foot. We just don't have enough room in this narrative to cover every street. I especially like looking around in this part of Dubuque to see how the tiers of houses have created a jumble of one house on top of another that almost looks like a pile.

Continuing with our walk on Montrose Terrace, the street follows the natural curvature of the bluff face and will soon curve to north. Almost immediately after the curve there will be an opening in the limestone block wall on the right-hand side that has a stairway coming up from Bluff Street.

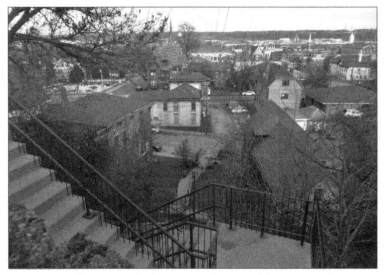

Bluff Street to Montrose Terrace Steps

Bluff Street to Montrose Terrace Steps

The stairway from Bluff Street to Montrose Terrace has 87 steps and makes several turns from Montrose down to where it meets Bluff Street just south of 15th Street at the edge of Dubuque's Jackson Park Historic District. The steps are very attractive and in great repair.

From the bottom, the stairway begins in a small park-like setting at the base of the bluff between 1461 and 1491 Bluff Street. The initial part of the stairway is more like a sidewalk with a few set of steps. The sidewalk becomes more stairway-like when it gets closer to the bluff. At that point it zig-zags along the side of the bluff. When the stairway reaches the large limestone block retaining wall, it is then supported by very attractive concrete pillars with a fluted design. The overall effect makes for a very pleasant climb or descent.

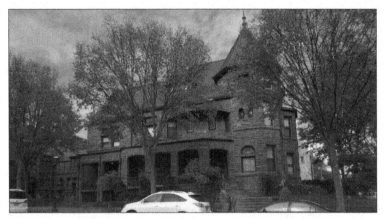

The Frank D. Stout house

Concluding the Tour and Returning to Our Starting Point

Our next Dubuque tour (Chapter 7) will begin from right here at the base of the Bluff Street to Montrose Terrace Steps. If you want to save that tour for another day, you can follow Bluff Street south back to our starting point at 11th and Bluff Streets next to the library. Needless to say there won't be a shortage of historic buildings to catch your attention on your walk back.

One building that caught my attention is at 1335-37 Bluff Street (on the west side of the street). It's a circa-1865 Italianate-style building with a cupola on top. Rather than being a brick or frame structure, this one is made out of stone. Another building that caught my eye is on the north side of 11th Street right across from the library. The house was built by the same man who donated the land for the library, Frank D. Stout. It's an enormous circa-1890 Richardsonian Romanesque red sandstone house. The intricate details of the house are amazing!

And I'm sure there will be plenty of other items catching your attention as you wrap up your tour.

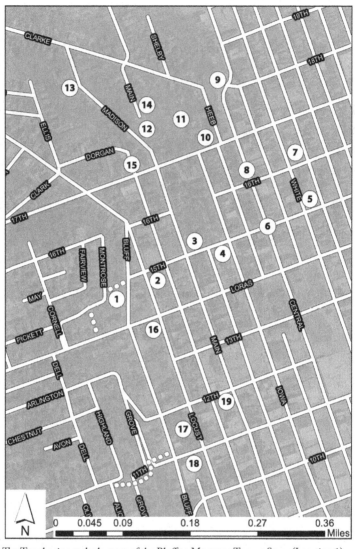

The Tour begins at the bottom of the Bluff to Montrose Terrace Steps (Location 1). All location references are numbers in circles. Dotted lines are pedestrian passages.

1. Bluff to Montrose Terrace Steps
2. Richards House
3. Jackson Park
4. St. Patrick's Church
5. St. Mary's Church/Steeple Square
6. 15th and Central – Great Murals and Buildings
7. 1651 White Street
8. Great Murals on Central
9. Old Firehouse
10. Old Seminary Building at 75 West 17th Street
11. Seminary Hill
12. Madison Street Retaining Wall and Private Stairway
13. 1921 Madison Street
14. Madison Park
15. Green Alley
16. Ryan House
17. 1145 Locust Street
18. Carnegie-Stout Public Library
19. Stained Glass Windows at St. Luke's Methodist Church

Chapter Seven

Exploring Dubuque's Neighborhoods at the Base of the Bluff

This tour explores the neighborhoods below the bluffs of Dubuque from Madison Park on the north to 11th Street on the south. The tour could be called exploring the greater Jackson Park area of Dubuque. Along the way we'll see wonderful homes, 19th-century commercial buildings with fabulous details, incredible murals, and many other surprises! This walk is a great opportunity to see the many layers of Dubuque's urban development.

This tour begins where the 11th Street walk (Chapter 6) ended at the bottom of the Bluff Street to Montrose Terrace Steps just south of 15th Street. This tour will wander around the streets in the area and end where the 11th Street walk began at the Carnegie-Stout Library at 11th and Bluff Streets.

Walking East on 15th Street

We'll start the tour by walking a few feet north from the bottom of the stairway to 15th Street and then turn right to head east on 15th Street. Almost immediately we'll run into the spectacular Richards House Bed and Breakfast at the southeast corner of 15th and Locust Streets.

Richards House

The circa-1883 house at 1492 Locust Street is now an inn and at the time of this writing was going under significant exterior renovation.

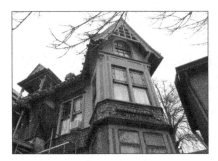

The Richards House

But based upon what has been completed, the final color palette and details will be fantastic. In a community with an abundance of amazing and whimsical 19th-century homes, this one, like many others, has to be near the top of the list. From the outside, the house is a collection of wood trims, shingles, and gables pointing in every direction imaginable. If you can get a good view, you'll see that the whimsical designs extend all the way to the top of the roof. If the inside is anything like the outside, it may be worthwhile to spend a night there.

Our walk continues east on 15th Street. After crossing Locust Street, 15th Street will become a red brick street for the next block. The next cross street is Main Street. The southwest corner of the intersection has a large 19th-century home that is now a funeral home. Jackson Park is at the northeast corner of the intersection. We'll keep walking east to the next cross street, Iowa Street.

Two Catholic Churches Within a Long Fly Ball of Each Other

St. Patrick's Catholic Church is at the southwest corner of 15th and Iowa Streets. The church is fine, but of much greater interest is to look ahead and see that there is another church with a very tall steeple less than an eighth of a mile away. That building, too, was a Catholic church called St. Mary's, and for many years it was active at the same time as St. Patrick's.

St. Mary's is now closed, and the church property has been renovated and repurposed into a combination of affordable housing,

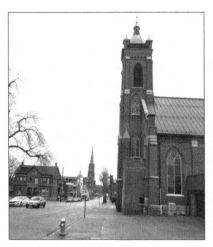
The two churches

child care center, community service facility, and multi-purpose event space. The property is now called Steeple Square.

In the late 19th century and early 20th century it was not uncommon for urban centers to have multiple Catholic churches within very close proximity of each other. They were usually built near each other to serve different ethnic or immigrant communities. In the case of 19th century Dubuque, Irish and Germans were the two predominant immigrant ethnic groups. Had there been another large ethnic group in Dubuque, we might have had a third Catholic church within our view. In the case of these two churches, St. Patrick's served an Irish community while St. Mary's served a German community. Whether intentional or by happenstance, providing an immigrant ethnic group their own church did help that group assimilate into their new country.

Standing on the Corner of 15th and Central

After checking out the two churches, our next major cross street will be Central Avenue. Central Avenue is amazing. It has great 19th-century commercial structures. Many of them have been exquisitely renovated. And it has murals. Really spectacular murals! As mentioned in the previous chapter exuberant murals are a recent addition to Dubuque's streetscape. They are a perfect complement to the abundance of 19th-century buildings and have brought new life to the street.

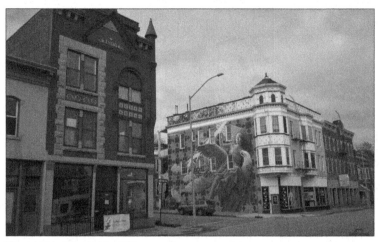

West side of Central at 15th

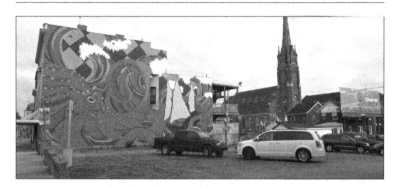

East side of Central south of 15th

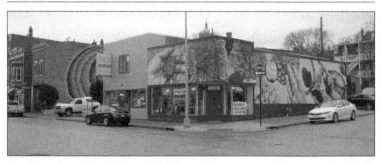

Southwest corner of 16th and Central

If you just stand at the intersection of 15th and Central and look around, you'll see something amazing in every direction. To our left on the northwest corner there is a mural covering all three stories of a storefront building in various shades of pink and blue of a woman riding on the back of a flying eagle. If we look across the street at the northeast corner, there is another predominately blue mural covering the entire side of the building of a person being engulfed by or transitioning into an owl. And on the southwest corner there is a meticulously restored circa-1890 storefront building. The details and brickwork on the building are amazing.

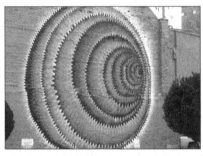

Central south of 16th

To find something amazing for the southeast corner of the 15th and Central intersection, we'll turn right and walk south on Central for less than half a block. There is a parking lot on the east side of Central right after the third building. If you turn around to look at the south wall of the third building (on the north side of the parking lot) you'll see a colorful mural of a giant orange-colored squid in a turbulent sea. The mural covers the entire wall, and, if you get the angle right, you can get both the mural and old St. Mary's church with its tall steeple into your photo.

The intersection of 15th and Central is also the midpoint between St. Patrick's and St. Mary's. Both of them are only a fly ball away from the intersection. If you would like to get a closer look of St. Mary's, now called Steeple Square, you can continue east on 15th Street to the next cross street (White Street). While on White Street there is a very interesting Second Empire-style 1891 brick building north of Steeple Square at 1651 White Street. The cream with green

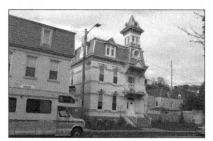

1651 White Street

trim building with a yellowish-ocher roof began as a single family home. It was later bought by St. Mary's to use as a school. The building is now multi-family housing.

To check out some more murals, we'll head north from the 15th and Central intersection. Before reaching 16th Street, there will be a parking lot on the west side of the street. Be sure to turn around to look at the wall on the south side of the parking lot. You'll see a vibrant almost psychedelic art-like mural covering the entire wall. When you reach 16th Street, you'll see a pawn shop at the southwest corner of the intersection with a mural-like sign on its front. If you look around the corner at the north side of the pawn shop, you'll see that the mural continues to cover almost all of the north wall.

But it's not just murals along Central Avenue. The 19th-century buildings all have details worth checking out. The building on the southeast corner of the Central and 16th intersection has a very interesting triple peaked roofline. The two-story building on the northwest corner has a very interesting logo of intertwined initials at the center of its roofline. It would be interesting know what the initials mean. One the great things about exploring is finding something that you have to do more research to figure out what it means.

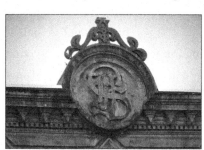

Logo at the NW of 16th and Central

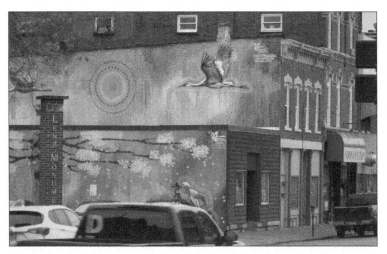

Mural on Central between 16th and 17th

But if we cross 16th street and keep walking north, we'll find a two-story mural split between two separate buildings on the east side of Central on the south side of the parking lot for Lenz Monument. It's a pastel colored mural of blossoms and flying cranes.

When we reach 17th Street, there will be a couple of steps on the west side of the street to get us down from the sidewalk to the

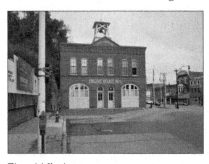

The old firehouse

street. If you look ahead to the north where Central Ave jogs to the right, you'll see the old 19th-century firehouse straight ahead. Up until a few years ago there was a stairway next to the firehouse connecting Central with Heeb Street up above. There are also two very interesting storefront buildings with intricate details at the northeast corner of the Central and 17th Street intersection. If you wish to continue north on Central, you will pass many more great buildings. But for our narrative we'll turn west (left) on 17th Street.

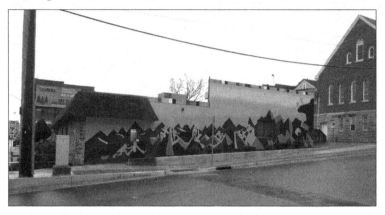

Southwest corner of 17th and Central

17th Street

When you turn left and head west on 17th Street, there will be another mural on the north wall of the building at the corner. This multi-colored mural is an imaginative abstract interpretation of children playing on mountains. As you continue west on 17th Street, you'll notice a very large building on the north side of the street and a bit up on the bluff. With the battlements on the top of its two towers it looks like it could be a fort or a castle.

The building at 75 West 17th was built in the 1850s as a women's seminary (college). The bluff behind the seminary building is called Seminary Hill. Later on the building became a theological seminary, a nursing home, and then a prayer center. The building was recently sold, and the new owners intend to renovate the building into apartments.

At this point, the north side of 17th Street is at the base of the bluff (Seminary Hill). As we continue walking along 17th, we'll be able to see houses higher up on the bluff and plenty of churches

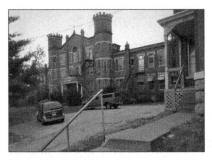

The old Seminary building

and interesting homes to check out on 17th Street. For purposes of this narrative, we'll continue walking to Madison Street. It will be the first street to actually cross 17th Street.

Madison Street

We'll turn right and head north on Madison Street. Very soon we'll run into a massive Dubuque-style retaining wall made out of large limestone blocks and a stairway at the end of the sidewalk. The stairway is privately owned and leads up to the house located above the retaining wall. At one time there was a public stairway at this location that went all the way to Madison Park at the top of the bluff. Forty some years ago there was a proposal to rebuild the steps. Unfortunately the proposal was not able to get enough traction to be acted upon favorably.

Being at the top of the bluff, Madison Park has great views overlooking Dubuque. If you want to check out the view, you can follow Madison Street up to the top of the hill; turn right on Clarke Drive; and then turn right again at Main Street. Main Street like so many other streets in this part of Dubuque also has great houses to check out. The park is at the end of Main Street. As you can see, a stairway would have been a great shortcut to the top.

Even if you do not want to check out Madison Park, a walk up Madison Street is worthwhile for at least part of the way as there are great retaining walls on the west side of the street and a fabulous circa-1893 Queen Anne-style home at 1921 Madison Street. The house almost looks like it's perched on the edge of a cliff. Can you imagine the views from inside the house?

Dorgan Place

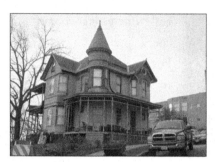

1921 Madison Street

Returning to 17th Street, we'll cross Madison Street and continue west. Almost immediately to our right will be Dorgan Place. In many ways Dorgan is more of an alley than a street. The most interesting thing about Dorgan is its pavement. It has a permeable surface and is called a "Green Alley." The permeable surface is designed to allow rain water to sink into the ground rather than run off into the street. Green Alleys are part of the Bee Branch Watershed flood control project. The Bee Branch Watershed project is discussed in greater detail in Chapter 8.

Dorgan Place loops behind the buildings on 17th Street and ends at the junction of Ellis Street and West Locust Street. We'll turn left to head south. The circa-1880s/90s house at the northeast corner of Locust and 17th Streets (395 West 17th Street) has many interesting architectural details worth investigating. For our tour, we'll cross 17th Street and continue south on Locust.

Locust Street

There is no shortage of interesting 19th-century buildings along Locust. When we reach 15th Street, we'll be passing the Richards House again. At the next cross street, Loras Boulevard, there are two houses side by side facing Locust at the southwest corner of the intersection at 1389 and 1375 Locust Street. Both of them were built in the 1870s. The house at 1389 Locust was built by William "Hog" Ryan after he moved from Galena (see Chapter 3) to Dubuque to open a meat packing plant. When he remarried after his first wife

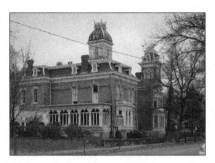

The Ryan House(s)

died he bought the house next door at 1375 Locust so that each of his families would have a house. The houses are collectively referred to as The Ryan House and have had different uses over the years including one as a restaurant.

After checking out the Ryan House we'll continue walking south on Locust. And again there will be plenty of nice buildings. When we cross 12th Street, there will soon be an amazing Queen Anne-style house at 1145 Locust Street on the west side of the street. Immediately south of the Queen Anne is a huge red sandstone house at 1105 Locust (see Chapter 6). Both houses were built in 1890s by members of the Stout lumber family.

With that we've reached 11th Street and the Carnegie-Stout Library where we started our 11th Street tour. If you want to check out some stained glass windows, you can turn left on 11th Street and walk east to Main Street (the next street) and then turn left again to walk back up to 12th Street.

St. Luke's Methodist Church at the southwest corner of 12th and Main has stained glass windows made by the Louis Comfort Tiffany Studios. You can see the windows from the outside, but they have a much greater impact when viewed from the inside. The windows were created between 1893 to 1931. The church's windows are one of the largest remaining collections of Tiffany stained glass.

With this our tour at the base of the bluff is finished. However, please feel free to keep on exploring as Dubuque has many more corners worth checking out.

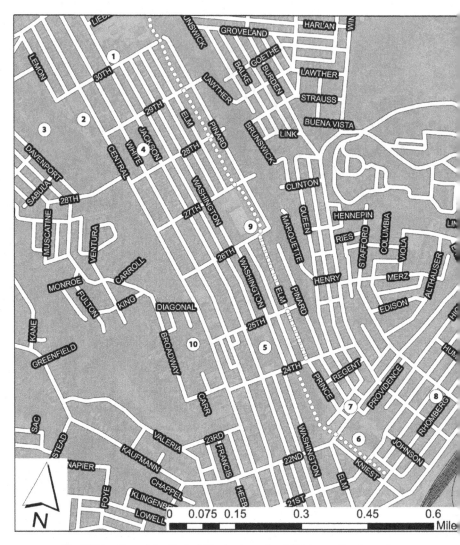

The Walking Tour of the Couler Valley begins at the old Dubuque Brewing and Malting Company Building at the northeast corner of 30th and Jackson Streets (Location 1). All location references are numbers in circles. The dotted lines are pedestrian passages.

1. Dubuque Brewing and Malting Company Building
2. Holy Ghost Church
3. ReEvolution Farmstead
4. Convivium Urban Farmstead
5. Comiskey Park
6. Bee Branch Creek Greenway
7. Mural and Restaurant at 609 East 22nd Street
8. Cremer's Meats at 731 East Rhomberg Avenue
9. Iowa Heritage Trail
10. Broadway Street Neighborhood Conservation District

Chapter Eight

Wandering Around Dubuque's North End in the Couler Valley

This walk explores Dubuque's North End neighborhood in the Couler Valley. Along the way we'll pass an old brewery, a grotto, two urban farms, some baseball history, a "daylighted" creek, another mural, a local taste sensation, an old railroad, several more 19th-century buildings, and some mysteries in the bluff. In short, the Couler Valley is the ideal place for a wandering adventure!

If you look closely at a topo map of Dubuque, you'll notice a flat-bottom valley, maybe at best a half-mile wide, splitting the bluffs that surround the flat riverside areas of Dubuque. The valley angles slightly to the northwest from downtown Dubuque and is called the Couler Valley. The Little Maquoketa River once flowed through the valley until it carved a shorter path to the Mississippi in an earlier geologic epoch.

As Dubuque grew, development on the North End of town pushed into the Couler Valley at a time when people still got around on foot or by public transportation (streetcars). Although it does not have the public stairways or the ornate houses as our other Dubuque walks, the North End of Dubuque does have a sufficient mass of buildings and a grid pattern of streets to make it an extraordinary area to explore on foot. The valley setting with bluffs on either side provides a nice contained space for a wandering adventure.

A good place to start our Couler Valley walk is at the intersection of East 30th Street and Jackson Street where the 1895-96-era Dubuque Brewing and Malting Company building is located at the northeast corner.

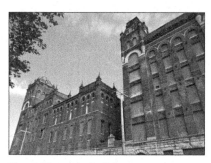

The old brewery building

Dubuque Brewing and Malting Company Building

When the Dubuque Brewing Company building was built in 1895-96, it was one of the largest breweries in the Midwest. Unfortunately, it was not able to survive Prohibition. Since then the building has had several other commercial and industrial uses. There are proposals for redevelopment, but as of right now the fate of the building is uncertain. The building had been proposed for listing on the National Register of Historic Places but was removed from consideration at the request of the owners.

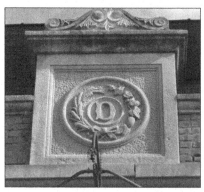

Old brewery buildings, and this one is no exception, are very interesting to check out as they usually have castle/ fortress-like features with great details in the brickwork to examine. This brewery has multiple tower-like details at the top, brick arches over the windows, and a stylized "D" over the center entrance. Dubuque has another old brewery building, the Dubuque Star Brewery, that is in much better shape than this one.

It is about two and a half miles to the south, east of downtown, and very close to the river.

The façade of the Dubuque Star Brewery building that we see today dates back to 1898. There are older building components withing the brewery complex behind the façade. Unlike the Dubuque Brewing Company, the Dubuque Star Brewery did emerge from Prohibition and regularly brewed beer until the 1980s. After that it went through a period of start and stop operations until it was finally shut down for good. The building has since been renovated and is now Stone Cliff Winery and Restaurant. The Dubuque Star name is still prominently displayed across the front and the building is on the National Register of Historic Places.

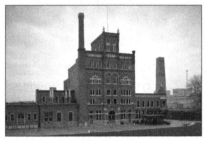

Dubuque Star Brewing building

If you go down to the riverside to check out the Dubuque Star Brewery building, you'll find a very nice walkway along the river called the Riverwalk. It connects the Star Brewery with the National Mississippi River Museum and Aquarium and has several outdoor art works along the way. The museum is a great attraction and well worth a visit. You can also check out the nearby old Shot Tower and watch trains cross the Mississippi River when you're down at the Dubuque Star Brewery building.

If you are interested in checking out other old brewery buildings, Wisconsin just over the river from Dubuque is the place go. At one time almost every Wisconsin town with a decent sized population had a small brewery along the lines of Dubuque Star Brewery. Over time, most them shut down as larger brands gobbled up market share. Ironically with the rise of craft beers, brew pubs, and micro-breweries, it is now the larger brands that are losing market share and feeling financial pressure.

In Potosi, Wisconsin (only a 26 mile drive from Dubuque and with a population of around 700) their small brewery opened in 1852 and shut down in 1972. After being dark for over thirty years, a community lead effort restored the brewery building and brought it back to life in 2008 as a micro/craft brewery and beer museum. The Potosi Brewery is now the town's largest attraction and brings in tens of thousands of visitors annually.

Exploring a Neighborhood on Foot

Rather than follow a fixed route with detailed right turn and left turn instructions, you may find it better when exploring an urban neighborhood like Dubuque's North End to adopt the mindset of wandering. Wandering is about letting yourself see (being mindful), and then letting what you see (or hear) guide you on where you go next. Adopting a wandering mindset can make every walk an adventure.

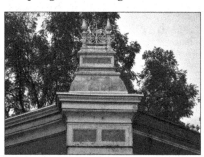

Architectural detail at 26th and Central

As you walk through the neighborhood south of the old Dubuque Brewing Company building you might notice that many of the houses are very similar. They tend to be simple gable-fronted frame structures that a worker could afford to buy or rent. As you continue walking, you may start to spot differences. Some homes may have been imaginatively remodeled or decorated; some brick buildings may have a faded advertising message from an earlier era; while another brick building might have a vibrant mural; and another might have a unique architectural feature that will cause you to stop and examine it. You may even notice which buildings were probably stores. Before everyone had a car, a working person's neighborhood had stores, taverns, and other services within easy walking distance.

It was while walking south from the Dubuque Brewing Company building that I started to hear the sound of church bells coming from the direction of Holy Ghost Church on Central Avenue. The songs were a wonderful addition to an already peaceful walk. And with that I started heading toward the bells to see what I could discover around the church.

Holy Ghost Church

The Holy Ghost Church complex is between 29th and 30th Streets. It is at the base of the bluff on the west side of Central Avenue. Central is only two streets west of Jackson Street where the old brewery building is located. Several of the Holy Ghost church buildings have recently been added to the National Register of Historic Places. The older building to the south was built around the same time as the brewery was built. The Italian Renaissance-style church with the tall bell tower in back was opened in 1916.

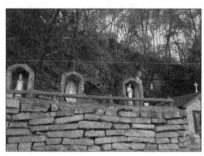

The church is fine but if you go around to the backside of the church you'll find an amazing grotto complex with the stations of the cross and a line of statues set into the side of the bluff. Statues include the Infant Jesus of Prague, the Virgin of Guadalupe, Saint Francis of Assisi, Jesus, and many others. It's almost like an All-Star batting line-up. Higher up on the bluff is a white statue of Mary looking down on everyone else.

Statues behind Holy Ghost Church

While near the bluffs in Dubuque, you might want to poke around to see what you can find without trespassing onto private property. With Dubuque getting its start as a lead mining center, you might find a now-gated mine entrance. Another possibility is finding the remains of an old brewery cave or even an old root cellar. Before refrigeration, caves and root cellars were dug to keep perishable items cool if not cold during the summer. Or you could stumble into something that is complete mystery. Running into mysteries is a big part of wandering.

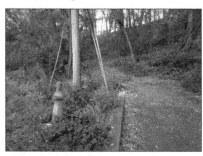

St. Francis and the path

With my wandering hat on I followed the base of the bluff north from the grotto. Before reaching the church school immediately to the north of the church, I ran into a beat up old paved pathway with a small statue of St. Francis at its opening heading up toward the top of the bluff. The pathway is technically on church-owned property so it is not a public right-of-way. But it doesn't matter as the path is impassible due to several fallen trees.

The pathway if it were passible connects to the church school's former ballfield above the bluff. The church sold the athletic field to ReEvolution Farmstead in 2018. At the time of this writing ReEvolution is still very much in its infancy and formative stage. So far, the south end of the athletic field has been converted into an urban farm. ReEvolution intends to make the entire property a sustainable urban farm open to community gardeners, market gardeners in need of additional growing space, and themselves to grow food for their own goal of providing healthy food to schools, hospitals, and grocery stores.

As part of their commitment to healthy food, ReEvolution is partnering on a hydroponics gardening effort at Convivium Urban Farmstead. Convivium is just east of the ReEvolution property and down below in the valley at 2811 Jackson Street (one and a half blocks south of the old brewery).

Convivium Urban Farmstead

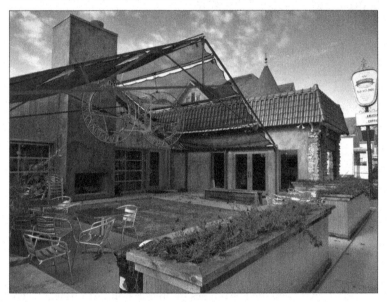

Convivium Urban Farmstead is amazing! It's a coffee shop, restaurant, art space, event space, performance space, kitchen space, classroom space, urban farm, and you name it, all located in a repurposed florist and greenhouse complex. Convivium's intent is to build a sustainable community around food. The exterior and interior design elements of Convivium are very contemporary, artistic, and nice. The interior wall of the event room even has a full size mural. They also offer classes and tours of the complex.

With food being the driving force at Convivium, every available square inch of the property is used to grow it. With its growing

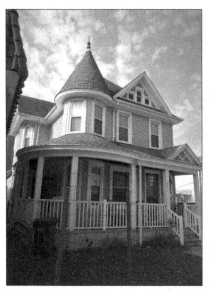
Sears Catalog House

capacity exceeded, Convivium has expanded its gardening/ urban farming activities into the back and side yards of many of its neighbors. As you continue your walk through the neighborhood you may want to keep an eye out for a Convivium garden plot.

The house immediately north of Convivium at 2813 Jackson is another very interesting curiosity. It is believed to be a Sears Catalog House. Between 1908 and 1940 it was possible to buy a house from the Sears Modern Home Catalog. A buyer would select a home from the catalog; choose a few options; and Sears would then ship all the necessary precut and fitted materials for assembling the house to the buyer by rail. The buyer (or the buyer's contractor) would then follow the provided instructions to put the house together. The advantages of buying home from Sears were that the precut and fitted materials would save building time and the economies of scale of manufacturing homes in a central location would save money.

You are welcome to go in any direction you choose from Convivium, but if you're a Chicago White Sox fan, you'll probably want to walk three and a half blocks further south on Jackson Street to 25th Street. There you'll find Dubuque's Comiskey Park at the southeast corner of Jackson and 25th Streets.

Dubuque's Comiskey Park

One hundred years ago, this was the site of Dubuque's minor league baseball park. When the baseball team moved to another location

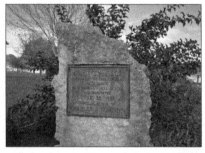

in Dubuque, the city acquired the property to use as a public park. Today you'll find a very nice neighborhood park with athletic fields, a playground, tennis courts, picnic tables, and a field house for indoor activities.

"Comiskey Field" monument

But the real reason for including the park in this book is found one block further south at the northeast corner of Jackson and 24th Streets. There you'll find an upright stone with a plaque mounted on it dated June 20, 1929. It dedicates the park as a recreation center named "Comiskey Field" in honor of Charles A. Comiskey. This is the same Charles A. Comiskey who founded the Chicago White Sox in 1901 and built the original Comiskey Park in Chicago in 1910. Charles A. Comiskey played part of his early baseball career in Dubuque and periodically helped the Dubuque minor league team find suitable players and managers.

If you choose to walk east on 24th Street after taking in the Comiskey Park monument, you'll come upon the Bee Branch Greenway at the southeast corner of the park.

Bee Branch Creek Greenway

So far every place that we've explored in this part of the Couler Valley has been in the Bee Branch Watershed. At one time the watershed was drained by Bee Branch creek flowing into the Mississippi River. As Dubuque expanded north into the Bee Branch watershed, the creek was, over the course of several projects in the early part of the 20th Century, rerouted into various tunnels and sewers. This put the creek out of sight and somewhere under the streets of Dubuque.

This all was all fine and wonderful until there was a heavy rain. Because the Bee Branch tunnels did not have sufficient capacity to handle a heavy rain, area residents could expect a flash flood and a flooded basement anytime there was a very heavy rain. And needless to say, this resulted in severe damage to roads and property.

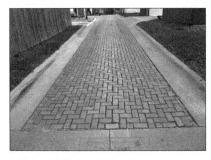
A "Green Alley"

With damage running into the millions if not tens of millions of dollars on a regular basis, the city decided that enough was enough and began a multifaceted program in the early part of this century to fix the problem. One of the facets was to build or enlarge retention basins above the bluffs to hold storm water rather than let it rush into the valley. Another was to rebuild the alleys in the basin area into "Green Alleys." That is, reconstructing the alleys with a permeable surface to allow storm water to slowly penetrate into the ground rather than rush into the street and eventually into the flood zone. Green Alleys are something that you might want to keep an eye out for as you wander around the Bee Branch basin. Dorgan Place which we explored in Chapter 7 is an example of a Green Alley.

The third facet, and one with several separate projects, was to "daylight" the creek. That is to get rid of the tunnels and return the creek to an outdoor channel with greatly increased carrying capacity. The Bee Branch Greenway which runs a little more than a third of a mile south from 24th Street (across from the southeast corner of

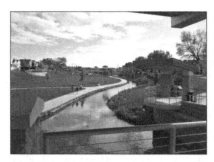

Bee Branch Creek Greenway

Comiskey Park) to Garfield Avenue is one of those projects.

Construction on the Bee Branch Greenway started in 2015 and finished in 2017. The Greenway has walking paths, playgrounds, benches, interpretive signs, an amphitheater, and very nice landscaping with wonderful design elements. The Greenway is a great way to continue your walk.

The first cross street that you'll reach after heading south on the Bee Branch Greenway is 22nd Street. If you are interested in murals, there is a great mural one block to east on the side of wonderful old brick building (609 East 22nd Street) that was once a neighborhood

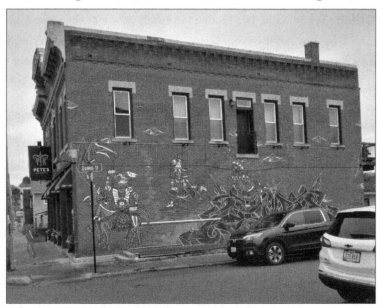

Mural at 609 East 22nd Street

market. The building now houses Pete's Thai Restaurant. If you've walked as far as Sacred Heart Church, you've gone too far. Just turn around and you'll see the mural.

As you continue south on the Bee Branch Greenway you'll soon reach Rhomberg Avenue. It's the last cross street before the end of the Greenway. If you're interested in a taste sensation that you are not likely to find elsewhere, you can walk three blocks east on Rhomberg to Cremer's Meats (731 Rhomberg Avenue) for a Turkey and Dressing sandwich.

Cremer's is a holdover from an era when people walked to their neighborhood market. One of their specialties is the Turkey and Dressing sandwich. Visualize turkey stuffing (or dressing, if you prefer) with chunks of turkey mixed into it and served on a small hamburger bun. If you're a fan of Thanksgiving and haven't had a turkey sensation in a while, you might want to walk the extra steps to try one.

With the end of the Bee Branch Greenway now very close, there are several ways to continue your Couler Valley wandering. One is to head back to our starting point with a walk along the Iowa Heritage Trail.

Iowa Heritage Trail

The Iowa Heritage Trail is a rail trail that follows the route of the former Chicago Great Western Railway from to Dubuque to Dyersville over 26 miles away. (Dyersville is where *Field of Dreams* was filmed and where you can still play catch on the ballfield featured in the movie.) The Great Western built the route in the 1880s (They had trackage rights to cross the Mississippi River on the Illinois Central bridge.) The Great Western was later acquired by the Chicago and North Western in 1968 who subsequently abandoned the route in 1981.

The Heritage Trail begins at the north end of the Bee Branch Greenway at 24th Street. When you get back to 24th Street just turn east. The bike trail is right there in the median of Elm Street. After two blocks of running in the median, the trail enters its own right-of-way at 26th Street. (The east bluff of the Couler Valley is just beyond the next street to the east.) From this point on the Heritage Trail is a very pleasant walk through a wooded park. It even runs behind the back-side of the old brewery where we started our wandering adventure in Dubuque's North End.

Because this is your wandering adventure, you can end it at any time. With the Heritage Trail running behind the old brewery, you could stop right here where you began. But if you want to continue your exploration, the "Broadway Street Neighborhood Conservation District" is nearby.

Broadway Street Neighborhood Conservation District

The Broadway Street Neighborhood Conservation District is on the west side of Central Avenue and runs from 24th Street on the south to Diagonal Street (between 25th and 26th Streets) on the north. The neighborhood is on a terrace above the Couler Valley but still well below the top of the bluff. A simple route to follow is to walk uphill on either West 24th Street or on Diagonal Street to Broadway Street. From there either go south to 24th or north to Diagonal and then return to Central Avenue. It's a relatively short loop that has several exceptional 19th-century buildings to make it interesting.

As for what is a "Conservation District," Dubuque has several Historic and Conservation Districts. A Historic District has a predominance of buildings of historic or architectural merit. Any exterior change to building in a Historic District that is visible to the public must go through a review and permitting process. A Conservation District has a lesser density of buildings of historic or architectural merit than a Historic District. A building cannot be demolished in a Conservation District without going through a review and permitting process.

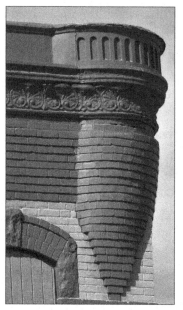

The "turret"

Some of the buildings in the Broadway neighborhood are contemporary, as in built sometime after World War II, and may not catch your attention. But what caught my attention is that many of the older 19th-century buildings have been carefully restored and have great vibrant colors. There are also buildings still in the restoration process, and it will be interesting to come back to check on their progress.

Some of the items that caught my attention in the neighborhood include the brick turret feature on the top corner of the commercial building on the northwest corner of Central and Diagonal. Another is a large 1850-era brick house at 2518 Broadway facing the street east of Broadway with a large metal star on its backside. Just to south of that building at 2500 Broadway is a large 1894-era Queen Anne-style home also decorated with a large star. And further south at the northeast corner of Broadway and 24th Street is an 1857-era house built out of irregularly shaped limestone blocks.

But the most intriguing item for me is the very attractive 1880 house with a mansard roof at the foot of Broadway right where it ends at 24th Street. The house has great details, colors, and the date of construction prominently featured above its middle window on the second floor. But if you look around to the west of the house toward the base of the bluff, you'll see what looks like an arched brick

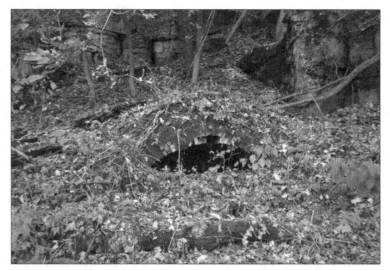

The mysterious "eyebrow"

eyebrow. It looks like a possible tunnel going into the bluff. You can see the eyebrow from the street, but don't go any closer as it is on private property.

The structure was probably a root cellar, but because it's off limits to examination and probably too dangerous to explore, it will probably remain a mystery. There certainly were lead mines and beer caves in the vicinity, so who knows for sure? Regardless of what it is, the brick eyebrow is a great example of what you can discover when you let your curiosity guide you on where you go in a wandering adventure.

And with this we'll end our Couler Valley adventure. But there is no reason why you can't keep going to see what else you can find!

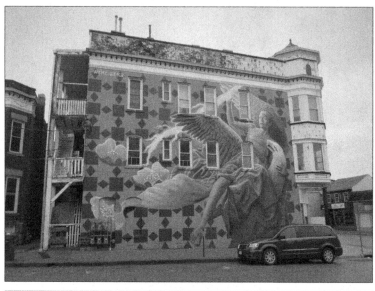

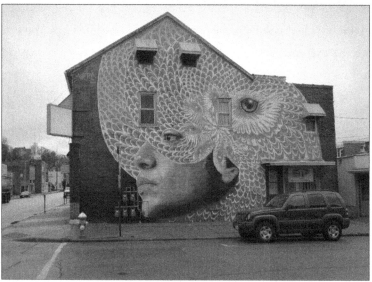

Murals at 15th and Central

Chapter Nine

Little Maquoketa River Mounds, Eagle Point Park, and the Julien Dubuque Monument

In this chapter we will climb some stairs to visit several Native-American mounds overlooking the Little Maquoketa River. We will then make a brief stop at Eagle Point Park to check out the view of the lock and dam down below on the Mississippi River. And finally we will go south of Dubuque for brief visit to Mines of Spain and climb some more stairs to check out the Julien Dubuque Monument and get another fantastic view of the Mississippi.

The Little Maquoketa River Mounds State Preserve is an island-like bluff with 32 Native-American ceremonial and burial mounds. The mounds are more than 160 feet above the Little Maquoketa River. The bluff is at the far north end of the Couler Valley and less than three miles from where we started our Couler Valley-Dubuque North End walk next to the old brewery in Chapter 8. The Preserve is easy to find as it is on the west side of U.S. Highway 52 (Central Avenue) and is identified by highway signs. If you drive over the Little Maquoketa River, you've gone too far.

The mounds were discovered in 1977 when the owner looked into developing the property. The State of Iowa bought the property in 1980 as a State Preserve to protect the mounds. The Preserve is managed by the Dubuque County Conservation Board. The Board in turn relies upon a Native-American council for guidance on how best to preserve the mounds as a sacred site.

As you drive up U.S. Highway 52, you may notice the relatively new overpass for the Iowa Heritage Rail Trail. The overpass allows the Heritage Trail to safely continue into the heart of Dubuque. The parking area for the mounds is very soon after the overpass. The approach trail to the mounds begins just beyond information kiosk at the edge of the parking area. The kiosk has a trail map and comprehensive background information on the mounds.

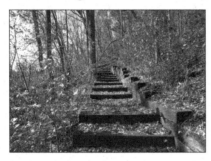

Steps to the mounds

The approach trail to the bluff can get a little marshy if there has been some rain, so you may have to do some hopping from dry spot to dry spot to get around the wet areas. Once you clear the low spots the trail winds its way through the woods to the top of the bluff with the assistance of a 120-step wood beam and dirt stairway.

Your climb through the woods is a perfect time to engage in the Japanese practice of *Shinrin-Yoku*, or "forest bathing." A forest bath is not a quick dip in a creek. It is more along the lines of breathing in the scents of the forest, being present, and walking quietly through the woods. Studies in Japan have shown that *Shinrin-Yoku* has significant health benefits, and many doctors in Japan are now prescribing *Shinrin-Yoku* for their patients.

As for the forest, when the mounds were built during the Middle and Late Woodland Period (more information on the Woodland Period and other phases of Native-American culture can be found in

Chapter 4), the bluff top was most likely a prairie savannah with very few trees and amazing views of the surrounding countryside. There is no doubt that the mounds were built here because of its commanding location.

The County Conservation Board would like to return the bluff top to a prairie savannah and has a program in place to remove the trees. Unfortunately, the last few years have been very wet and it has been a struggle to keep up with the forest growth. Trees can sometimes grow like weeds in a wet environment, so it may be some time before the bluff is restored to the state it was in when the mounds were built.

When you get near the top of the bluff there will a "Y" junction in the trail. It doesn't matter which direction you go since the trail loops together at the top. There are short extensions at each end of the loop. The northeast extension leads to an information kiosk with various Native-American blessings given during the dedication of the Preserve and to a very good overlook of the Little Maquoketa River at the base of the bluff. The view is best in the winter when the leaves are off the trees. While looking across the river valley you may see where the river abandoned the Couler Valley for a shorter route to the Mississippi.

Once on top of the bluff, the trail follows a substantial chain link fence that surrounds and protects the mounds. Helicopters were used to bring construction materials for the fence to the top of the bluff. Trees have since fallen on the fence to create gaps in the barrier. The Preserve's Native-American advisory council would like to see the fence removed to give the mounds a more open and natural feel. The County Conservation Board agrees and is trying to determine how best to accomplish this. It won't be easy because there is no way to get construction equipment to the top, so any removal work will have to be done by hand.

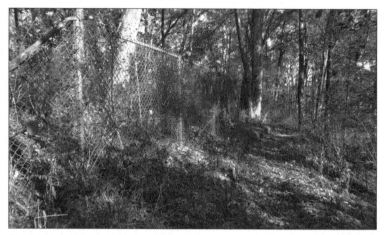

The fence and mounds

With so much overgrowth, it is not always easy to recognize the mounds on the other side of the fence, but if you give it some time and relax your eyes the shapes of the mounds on the other side of the fence will become more apparent. Removing the fence, trees, and overgrowth will go a long way in making it easier to appreciate the beauty and significance of the mounds. Until that happens you can go to Gramercy Park in East Dubuque (Chapter 4) to get a better sense of what Native-American mounds look like.

In the meantime the Little Maquoketa River Mounds Preserve is a very nice walk through the woods with a 120-step stairway thrown in as an added bonus.

Eagle Point Park

A trip to Dubuque would not be complete without a visit to Eagle Point Park. The view of the Mississippi River from high up on the bluff is wonderful. From the top you can see the hills of Wisconsin and Illinois on the other side of the river. Just to the south is the bridge to Wisconsin and directly below is the General Zebulon Pike

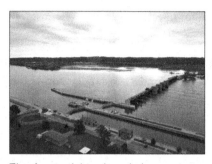

The river and dam down below

Lock and Dam. The dam was built during the 1930s to ensure that the river maintained a sufficient depth for navigation. And with the Mississippi River still a very active transportation corridor for bulk materials, you'll have a very good chance of seeing tow boats and barges passing through the lock and going up and down the river.

Eagle Point Park is Dubuque's largest city park and is open from May through October. The only downside is that dogs are not allowed in the park. To reach the park from the Little Maquoketa River Mounds Preserve, just take U.S. Highway 52 (Central Avenue) back into Dubuque. Turn east (left) when you reach Rhomberg Avenue. Turn left again at Shiras Avenue and proceed north to the Eagle Point Park gatehouse. There is a nominal fee to enter the park.

The park was built in the early part of the 20th century and was even served by streetcars. The Trolley Line Trail is a paved bike path that follows the former streetcar route into the park. During the 1930s the WPA (Works Progress Administration) built many new landscape features and pavilions under the direction of Park Superintendent Alfred Caldwell.

A fan of Frank Lloyd Wright, Caldwell had the new WPA structures and features built in Wright's famous Prairie School style. Dubuque does not have any Frank Lloyd Wright buildings, but when you walk around Eagle Point Park, you might think you're walking through an outdoor Frank Lloyd Wright exhibit. If you want to see more of Frank Lloyd Wright's creativity, you can visit Taliesin

(Wright's summer home and studio) in Spring Green, Wisconsin. It is less than 70 miles from Dubuque.

In the early years of Eagle Point Park there was a beach on the river and a stairway built into bluff to connect the park on top of the bluff with the beach down below. The beach was eliminated with the construction of the dam in the 1930s, and the stairway slowly fell into disrepair. The stairs were finally closed in the 1960s.

There may be portions of the old stairway somewhere on the bluff, but between the dam, a new bridge to Wisconsin, and other construction in the area, finding an orphan section or two of the stairway would be extremely difficult if not impossible. You can however get a good look at the geology of the area by checking out an old quarry at the bottom of the bluff.

To check out the old quarry, return to Rhomberg Avenue. When you reach Rhomberg, instead of heading to the center of Dubuque, turn left and take Rhomberg east to where it ends. The old quarry and the enormous vertical wall of limestone are to your left. Access to the base of the limestone wall may be difficult because most of the land in the area is privately owned. It doesn't matter because you can get a good idea of the geology right from the road.

But it would very cool if there still was a stairway that you could climb to reach the top.

Julien Dubuque Monument

The Julien Dubuque Monument is around four miles south of Dubuque in the Mines of Spain Recreation Area. Mines of Spain is 1400 acres of woods, bluffs, and creeks. It has a nature center, hiking trails, a canoe route, and plenty of places to explore. No attempt will be made in this narrative to describe them all.

To hike to the monument we'll park the car in the "canoe access" parking lot next to Catfish Creek. This is the same area where Julien

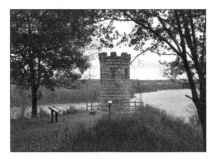

The Julien Dubuque Monument

Dubuque mined lead in 1788 when the land west of the Mississippi River was still nominally a Spanish possession. The hiking trail to the monument starts from the parking lot.

With the trail passing through the forest the entire way, this, like the Little Maquoketa River Mounds, is a perfect place for practicing *Shinrin-Yoku* or forest bathing. Many of the trees along the way are quite old and huge. Keep an eye out for huge burls on many of the trees.

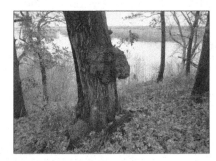

One of the many burls

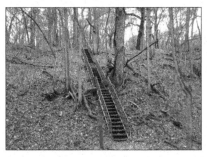

Stairs on the trail

Almost immediately after you start walking, you'll reach a metal stairway with 50 steps going up a steep portion of the bluff. From the top of the stairway the trail continues uphill and has an occasional wood beam and dirt step thrown in for good measure. At the top of the trail you'll run into the parking area at the end of the monument approach road. From there, just follow the path to the Julien Dubuque monument. There are several information signs on the area's history along the way.

The circular castle-like limestone monument was built in 1897 and is where Julien Dubuque is now buried. The views from the monument looking down on the Mississippi River are spectacular. There is a good chance of seeing tow boats and trains pass by at the same time. Those are the tracks of the Canadian Pacific Railway hugging the riverbank down below.

When you're ready, you can return to your car the same way you came up. Since the trail is less than a mile each way, this is a great way to approach the monument. It's also another opportunity to climb a stairway.

To reach the trailhead, take U.S. Highway 52 or 61 south from Dubuque. When you reach Grandview Avenue, get off the highway and go east to Julien Dubuque Drive and turn south. Julien Dubuque Drive is almost a frontage road for U.S. Highway 52/61. Julien Dubuque Drive will eventually curve to the east and intersect with Mines of Spain Road. Turn south on Mines of Spain Road. The road will curve to east and will soon reach the approach road to the monument. Stay on Mines of Spain Road as it curves south again for just a little bit more. The trailhead and parking lot will be on the left just before Mines of Spain Road crosses Catfish Creek.

• • •

With this, our tour of Galena and Dubuque is complete. By using this narrative as a starting point, I am sure you will make many more discoveries in this extraordinarily scenic and interesting part of the country.

How This Book Came To Be

Having grown up and spending most of my life in Chicago along with having significant Galena roots, I was already quite familiar with Galena and Dubuque. It was while I was considering a book on "wandering" that I ran into an article by Dan Koeppel in the September 2010 issue of *Backpacker Magazine* about climbing public stairways in Los Angeles. Intrigued by the concept of climbing public stairways as a vehicle to explore city neighborhoods, I went to Los Angeles soon after reading the article to find out first hand.

My trip to Los Angeles was amazing and it opened up a whole new dimension in my own personal hiking, exploration, and wandering endeavors. As a result, stairways became a big part of my 2012 book *The Gentle Art of Wandering* and one of the many ongoing themes in my wandering blog at www.gentleartofwandering.com.

With my new found appreciation of stairways, I was certain that communities in the Upper Mississippi River Valley must have stairways. So my dog Petey and I decided to go on a long road trip in 2013 from New Mexico, where we now live, to find out for sure. On our trip to the Upper Mississippi River Valley, we found and climbed public stairways in Dubuque, Galena, Alma (Wisconsin), Red Wing (Minnesota), Stillwater (Minnesota), St. Paul, and Minneapolis.

When we got back from our trip I wrote several different blog posts about those stairways. The blog posts on the stairways in Galena and especially Dubuque have proven to be very popular. More than six years since writing those blog posts people are still running across the posts and sharing them with their friends on social media. Finally, because of the many people who keep visiting the Galena and Dubuque blog posts, Petey and I decided that we should turn our explorations into a walking book on Galena and Dubuque.

With that, Petey and I made several trips to the Galena and Dubuque area in 2019 to do our research. We soon realized that there were not enough stairways in Galena and Dubuque to warrant a stairway specific book. But we did discover that there was plenty of material in the form of natural beauty, scenic views, history, wonderful buildings, interesting neighborhoods, and many other surprises for a great walking book. We believe that the combination of public stairways and the new material that we found makes both Galena and Dubuque extraordinary places to explore on foot!

We hope you agree, and that you'll get out and find way more than what we found.

Sources

The contents of this book are based upon the on-the-ground research conducted by my dog Petey and myself, knowledge that I already had, and from several sources that I consulted for background information. Sources include:

Ulysses S. Grant, *Personal Memoirs of U.S. Grant*. New York: Penguin Classics. 1885.

Ron Chernow, *Grant*. New York: Penguin Press. 2017.

Kenneth N. Owens, *Galena, Grant, and the Fortunes of War*. Dekalb, Illinois: Northern Illinois University. 1963.

Carl H. Johnston, Jr., *The Building of Galena: An Architectural Legacy*. 1977.

Steve Repp, *Ulysses S. Grant: The Galena Years*. 1994

Diann Marsh, *Galena, Illinois: A Brief History*. Charleston, S.C.: History Press. 2010.

Illinois State Geologic Survey, *Guidebook 42: Guide to the Geology,...*, *of the Driftless Area of Northwestern, Illinois, Jo Daviess County*. University of Illinois at Urbana Champaign. 2016

City of Galena, *Historic District Structure Database*. An online resource of the City of Dubuque website.

Dubuque County Historical Society, *Dubuque History Trail Tours*. This consists of five booklets on Dubuque's historic neighborhoods. They are available at the National Mississippi River Museum & Aquarium.

Lawrence J. Sommer, *The Heritage of Dubuque: An Architectural View.* First National Bank of Dubuque. 1975.

Randy Lyon, *Encyclopedia Dubuque.* An invaluable online resource for all things Dubuque.

Geologic Society of Iowa, *Guidebook 63: Geology in the Dubuque Area.* Iowa Department of Natural Resources, Des Moines, Iowa. 1997.

City of Dubuque, *Architecture and Historic Resource Reports.* There are several reports on Dubuque's historic neighborhoods available on the City of Dubuque website. The website also has surveys on individual historic properties.

Acknowledgements

Although all of the on-the-ground research and writing was done by me, I couldn't have finished this book without the help of many other people. To that end I want to thank all of the people who I met on my walks, the people I emailed, and the people who I called on the phone for answering my many questions on Galena and Dubuque. I especially want to thank Randy Lyon, Michael Gibson, and Steve Repp for providing me so much background information on Galena and Dubuque. Randy is the creator of *Encyclopedia Dubuque,* Michael is the director of the *Center for Dubuque History* at Loras College, and Steve is the "go to" person for Galena history.

I want to thank Mark Moran, the City Administrator of Galena, and Terry Renner, Mayor of Galena, for providing me information on Galena and its public stairways. I especially want to thank Mark Moran for providing the base map of Galena's streets. That data was essential for preparing the Galena map in this book.

I want to thank David Johnson and Jon Dienst with the City of Dubuque for the information they provided me on Dubuque's public stairways. And I especially want to thank Caleb Scheidel and Nikki Rosemeyer of the City of Dubuque's GIS Department for the base map of Dubuque's streets. Again, that data was essential for preparing the Dubuque maps in the book.

I want to thank Mark Sullivan for the design and the look and feel of the book. And I want to thank Jonathon Carlson for preparing the maps. I want to give special thanks to my wife Claudia for taking the time to review and correct the material in this book.

But most of all I want to thank my dog Petey who accompanied me on all of my research trips to Galena and Dubuque and for giving his approval to all of the tours described in this book.

About the Author

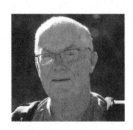 David Ryan left his conventional job in the business world at the age of 49 to rearrange his life into a mixture of income-producing and personal activities. Since making that change he has found time to walk the 2,180-mile Appalachian Trail, walk the Camino de Santiago from Le Puy in France to Santiago de Compostela in the far west of Spain, become involved in archaeology, earn a black belt in aikido, and pursue several outdoor and walking activities. He is the author of several walking books and writes a blog on walking, hiking and wandering at www.gentleartofwandering.com. David lives in Albuquerque, New Mexico with his wife Claudia, and his three dogs, Paddy, Petey, and Sparky. To contact David Ryan or to receive updates, please visit www.gentleartofwandering.com.

Author photo by Robert Browman/Albuquerque Journal